D1824858

THE
PARENTS'
EMERGENCY
GUIDE

Throughout the book we have referred to the child as "he" or "him" – obviously we do so only for convenience. Similarly, we often refer to the "parent" – by which we mean either the mother or father or any other person who may be acting, either temporarily or permanently, in a parental role.

CONSULTANTS

Dr. H. Ahluwalia (Medical support group – Boots Company Ltd.)

Dr. D. B. Garrioch (Consultant in Obstetrics and Gynaecology) Pembury Hospital.

M. Jennings (Obstetric physiotherapist) St. Thomas's Hospital, London.

Dr. Gwyneth Lewis (Medical Officer) Sussex University.

Dr. M. Modell (GP) The James Wigg Practice, London.

Miss. J. M. Redfern (SRN RSCN Pediatric Unit – Brook General Hospital)

Shirley Smith (Matron of North London Kindergarten)

Dr. M. K. Thompson (General Practitioner) Croydon, Surrey.

James A. Williams (Field Officer-Training, British Red Cross Society)

Family Planning Association

THE PARENTS' EMERGENCY GUIDE

An Action Handbook for Childhood Illnesses and Accidents

The Diagram Group

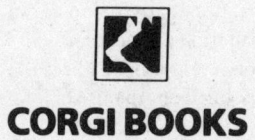

CORGI BOOKS

THE PARENTS' EMERGENCY GUIDE

A CORGI BOOK 0552 12740 X

First publication in Great Britain

PRINTING HISTORY

Corgi edition published 1986

Copyright © 1986 Diagram Visual Information Ltd.

This book is set in 9/11pt Baskerville

Corgi Books are published by Transworld Publishers Ltd.,
61–63 Uxbridge Road, Ealing, London W5 5SA, in Australia
by Transworld Publishers (Aust.) Pty. Ltd., 26 Harley
Crescent, Condell Park, NSW 2200, and in New Zealand by
Transworld Publishers (N.Z.) Ltd., Cnr. Moselle and
Waipareira Avenues, Henderson, Auckland.

Printed and bound in Great Britain by
Cox & Wyman Ltd, Reading

All rights reserved. No part of this book may be reproduced or
utilized in any form or by any means electronic or mechanical,
including photocopying, recording or by any information
storage and retrieval system without permission in writing from
the Publisher.

The nature of information on the treatment of accident or
illness is that it is constantly evolving and often subject to
interpretation. While the greatest efforts have been made to
ensure the accuracy and completeness of the information
presented, the reader is advised that no claim can be made that
all relevant information concerning the treatment of accident
or illness is included in this book. In addition, the reader
should note that this book is not a manual for self diagnosis or
self treatment, and that he is advised to consult his general
practitioner for information on, or treatment for, any medical
condition. Corgi Books cannot be held responsible for error or
any consequences arising from the use of information contained
herein.

Foreword

A new baby brings problems as well as joys and in the middle
of the night the smallest molehill of an illness can look like an
unscalable Everest to harassed parents. Doctors make due
allowance for parents' fears, but are apt to be less than patient
with those who bring their child to the surgery twice a week
with every transient snuffle. The Parents' Emergency Guide
will not only keep you from being your GP's least favourite
family but – more importantly – will help you to put your
offspring's ills in perspective and sleep a little more easily. Do
not regard it as a Holy Writ. Do not read through it at one
sitting like "War and Peace", but in an emergency, consult it as
you would an experienced friend. If the answer is simply not
there, get in touch with your family doctor and ask his advice –
a commodity more valuable in many cases than medicine. And
perhaps, when you have had a word with him, the problem will
no longer be an emergency at all.

Dr. Geoffrey Smerdon
M.A. (Oxon), B.M., B.Ch., M.F.O.M.(R.C.P.)

CONTENTS

Section 1:
ILLNESS

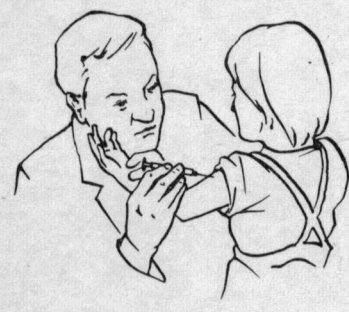
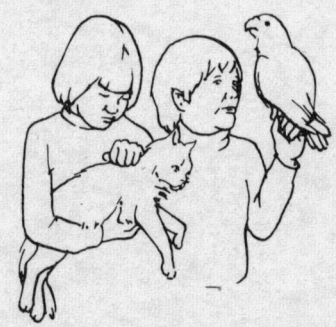

**EMERGENCY INDEX:
See page 127**

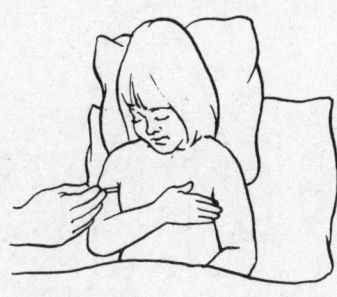
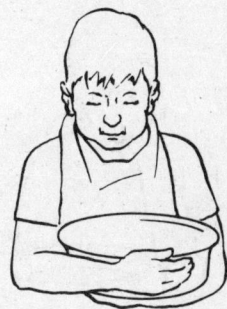

CONTENTS

Section 2: ACCIDENTS

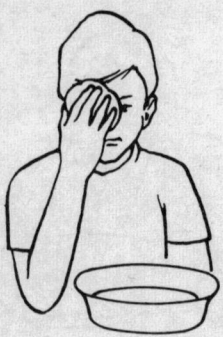

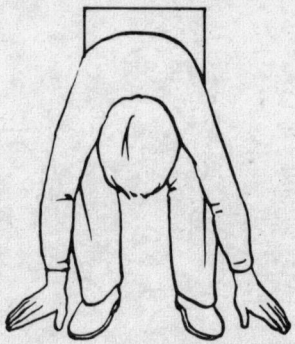

**EMERGENCY INDEX:
See page 127**

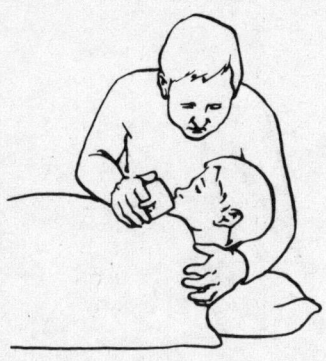

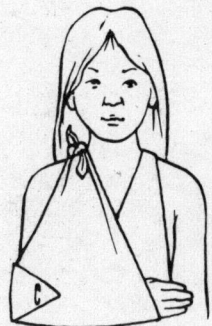

Section 1: ILLNESS

Introduction

How can you tell if your child is ill? This is not always easy,
particularly for parents today who are less likely than their
grandparents to have had the experience of large families and
numerous young relatives. For a new parent with a very young
baby even a sneeze can be worrying, while a harmless heat rash
can seem like the forerunner of a dangerous disease. Obviously,
with time, experience takes over. As a child grows he develops a
normal behaviour pattern and it is usually any sudden change
in this that makes a parent suspect sickness.
But there is a variety of illnesses that can occur during
childhood, and many of them have much the same symptoms.
Sweating, fever, and a high temperature may just be the
start of a cold; or they may indicate the onset of measles or
diphtheria. In order for treatment to occur promptly and
efficiently, it is important for parents to learn to recognize and
distinguish between the signs and symptoms of the more
common childhood complaints, to know how to cope with a
sick child and, above all, to know when to call the doctor. The
following pages give a comprehensive guide to illness in
childhood.

They explain what illness is, when and how it occurs, and explain how and why infection spreads. Also included is a comprehensive coverage of the common, and less common, disorders of childhood. These range from the common cold to the so-called 'childish complaints' such as measles, mumps, and chicken pox, and also include various digestive, respiratory, and other problems. There is also guidance on vaccinations. Information on coping with a sick child includes how to take a temperature, how to bring down a fever, and what sort of diet and amusements are recommended for a child convalescing from illness.

Illness of one kind or another is inevitable during childhood. But many preventive measures can and should be taken. A responsible attitude to vaccinations is essential. Despite current debate, it is vaccination that has turned former killers such as diphtheria, tetanus and polio into dormant diseases. In addition, hygiene, a good diet, plenty of exercise and rest are other commonsense measures that will ensure that your child has the best possible chance of fighting whatever illnesses may occur.

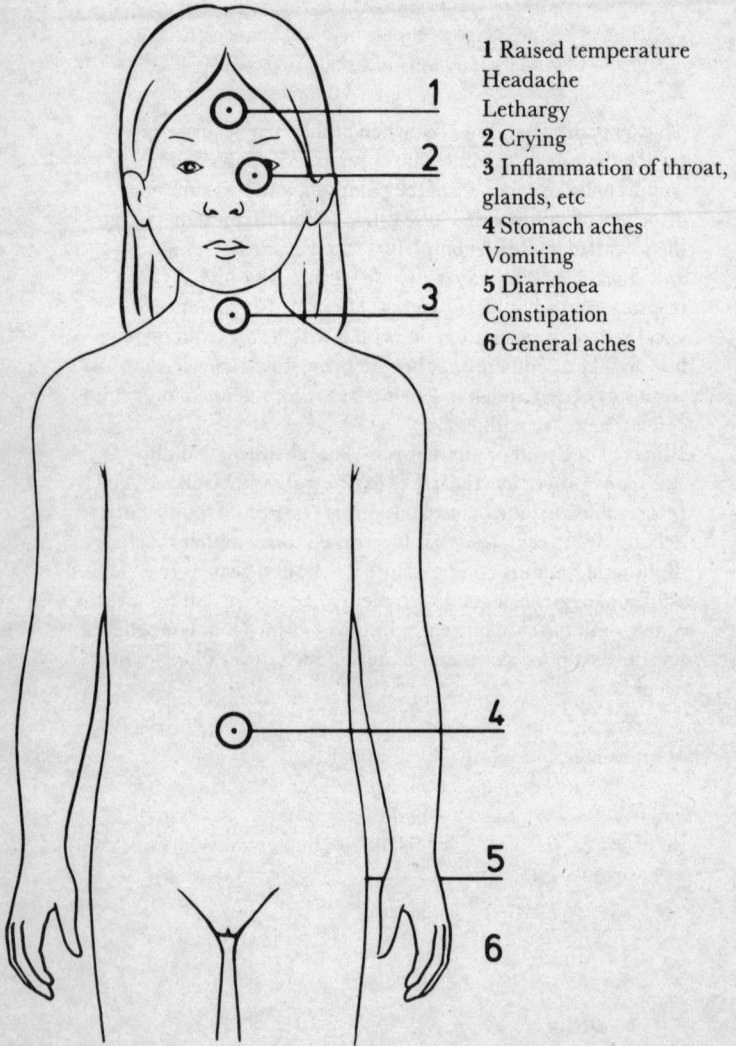

1 Raised temperature
Headache
Lethargy
2 Crying
3 Inflammation of throat, glands, etc
4 Stomach aches
Vomiting
5 Diarrhoea
Constipation
6 General aches

symptoms and signs

The onset of illness in children may be accompanied by disturbing symptoms and signs. Many result from poisons released by agents of infection in the body before its defences can crush them. In many infections a child sweats, shivers, runs a high temperature, and is tired, flushed, apathetic, and lacks appetite. Rashes or spots appear in scarlet fever, measles, and German measles. Diarrhoea and vomiting may stem from a variety of causes. Sore throats come with diphtheria, glandular fever, and poliomyelitis. Aching and shivering come with mumps, chicken pox, German measles, and stress. But many of these symptoms and signs can also have trivial causes and vanish overnight.

acute or chronic illness

Acute
An acute illness comes on suddenly, intensifies sharply, and usually lasts a short time. Such an illness is not necessarily serious – the common cold is a good example.

Chronic
A chronic illness is one that lasts for a considerable time without any rapid developments in the patient's condition. In a chronic infectious illness the unaided body is unable or slow to destroy the agent of infection. Most chronic illnesses, however, can be cured or helped by medical treatment. As with acute illnesses, the term chronic has no bearing on the severity of the disease or its symptoms.

the development of illness

Before birth
Some conditions are inherited: haemophilia and sickle-cell anaemia for instance. Others are acquired during foetal development or during birth, for instance some kinds of brain damage and deafness due to German measles in the pregnant mother. Both groups are termed congenital if present at birth. Other examples of congenital disorders include club foot, cleft palate, and various heart or digestive disorders. Many can be corrected with surgery or drugs.

In life
Most diseases arise during life. These include nutritional diseases; allergies; infestation of skin, hair, or internal organs by parasites; and infection of the body by disease microorganisms. Most infections result from hostile microorganisms entering the body through nose, mouth, ears, eyes, urogenital openings, or broken skin.

the causes of disease

1 Bacteria are microscopic one-celled organisms, some of which normally live harmlessly on skin, in the nose, mouth, throat, and lungs, and in intestines. Reduced bodily resistance allows some to multiply and cause sore throats or other ailments. Illness can occur if bacteria normally in one part of the body get into another. But most disease bacteria enter the body from outside. Diphtheria, scarlet fever, tuberculosis, and whooping cough are bacterial diseases.

2 Viruses are smaller than bacteria and live as parasites, active and reproducing only in other living cells, which they break down. Viral diseases include the common cold, chicken pox, influenza, measles, mumps, and smallpox.

3 Rickettsias are germs found in certain fleas, lice, mites, and ticks. Rickettsias cause serious diseases such as typhus.

4 Fungi are non-green plants. Tiny fungi cause ringworm and some lung diseases.

5 Protozoan parasites are one-celled animals some of which can get inside the body to cause diseases including amoebic dysentery, malaria, and sleeping sickness.

6 Metazoan (many-celled) parasites include tapeworms, roundworms, fleas, and lice.

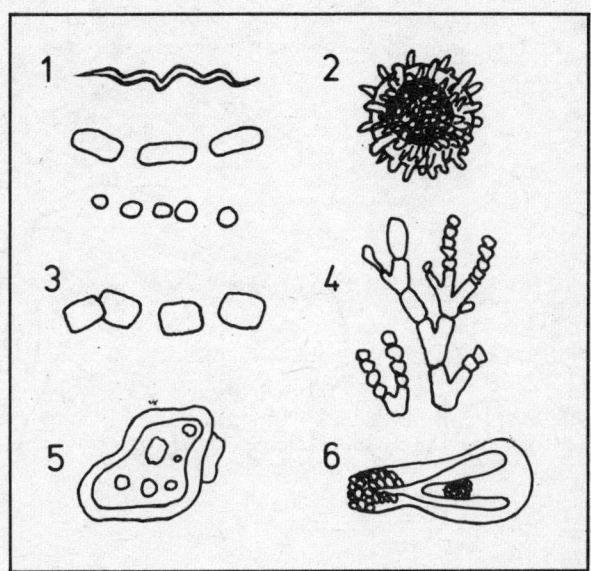

spreading of disease

1 Disease is often spread by bacteria or viruses airborne in droplets breathed, coughed, or sneezed out by infectious people and breathed in by others. (A sneeze can hurl 20,000 droplets 15ft; 4.6m.) People sometimes contract anthrax and tuberculosis by breathing in dusty air bearing old, dried bacterial spores.

2 Some skin conditions spread by skin-to-skin contact.

3 Infected soil or dust entering a cut can cause tetanus or gangrene.

4 Pets may harbour and transmit diseases. For example: dogs, tapeworms; parrots, psittacosis; guinea pigs, encephalitis; turtles, salmonella poisoning; horses, glanders; cattle, brucellosis; cats, toxoplasmosis; various mammals, rabies.

5 Food or water contaminated by germs at source, or by poor personal hygiene, can cause diseases such as brucellosis, cholera, typhoid, dysentery, and poliomyelitis.

6 Flies can infect food with bacteria if it is left uncovered.

7 Bites by parasitic insects can also transmit disease.

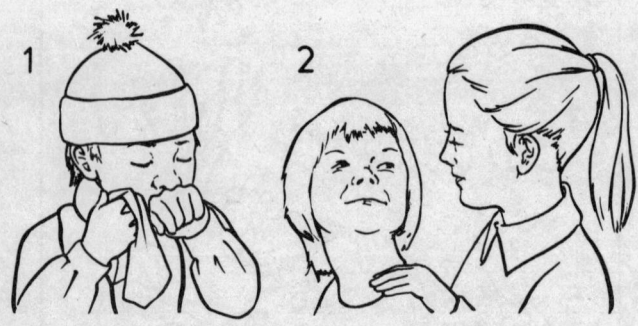

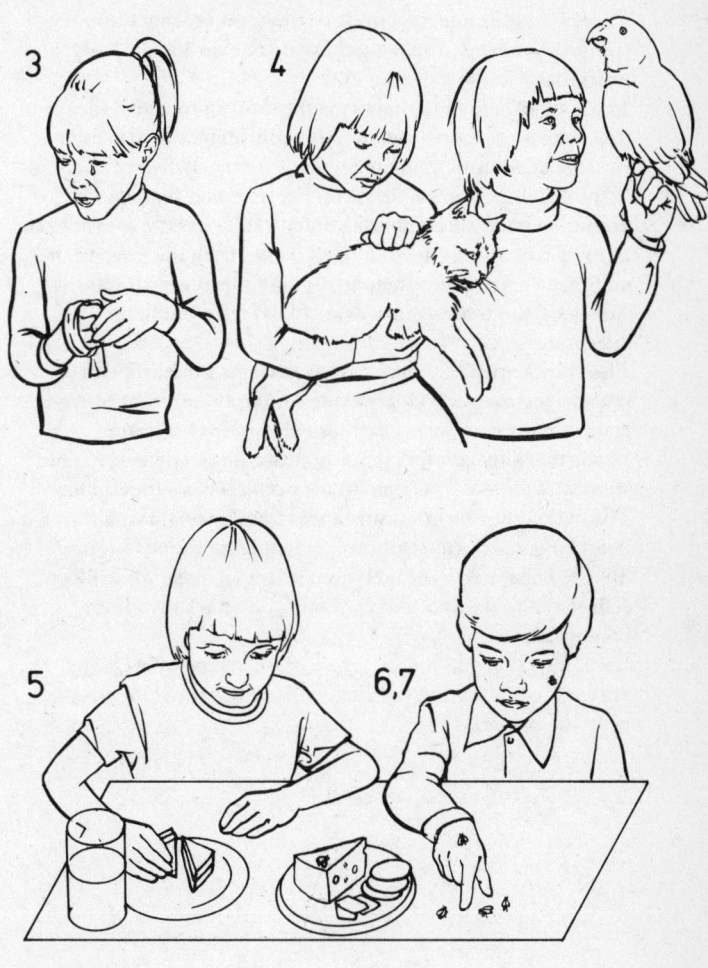

the body's safeguards

The body fights infection in three ways: preventing the entry of foreign organisms; attacking those that get inside the body; and neutralizing those it cannot kill.

The body's main outer barrier is the skin, a protective sheath that guards the tissues below. Also, antiseptic substances in sweat exuded from the skin kill many germs. Different openings in the skin have special defences. For instance, tear glands produce a bacteria-combating fluid that bathes the eyes at each blink. Tears also wash out foreign bodies from the eyes. In the mouth, salivary glands help to combat infectious substances. Adenoids and tonsils make white blood cells that fight infection.

The body's openings and internal passages are lined with mucous membranes. Coated with antiseptic substances in a layer of mucus, these act as physical barriers and traps.

Inside the body certain organs produce special defences. The stomach secretes acids that attack bacteria in swallowed food. The liver filters harmful substances from blood flowing through it, and creates clotting substances that help wounds heal. Spleen, bone marrow, and lymph nodes all make white blood cells that circulate around the body and attack invading organisms.

Local infection may trigger an increase in blood flow to the affected part, creating swelling, pain, and pus (white blood cells and bacteria).

1 Tear glands
2 Adenoids
3 Salivary glands
4 Tonsils
5 Lymph nodes
6 Mucous membranes
7 Liver
8 Spleen

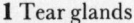

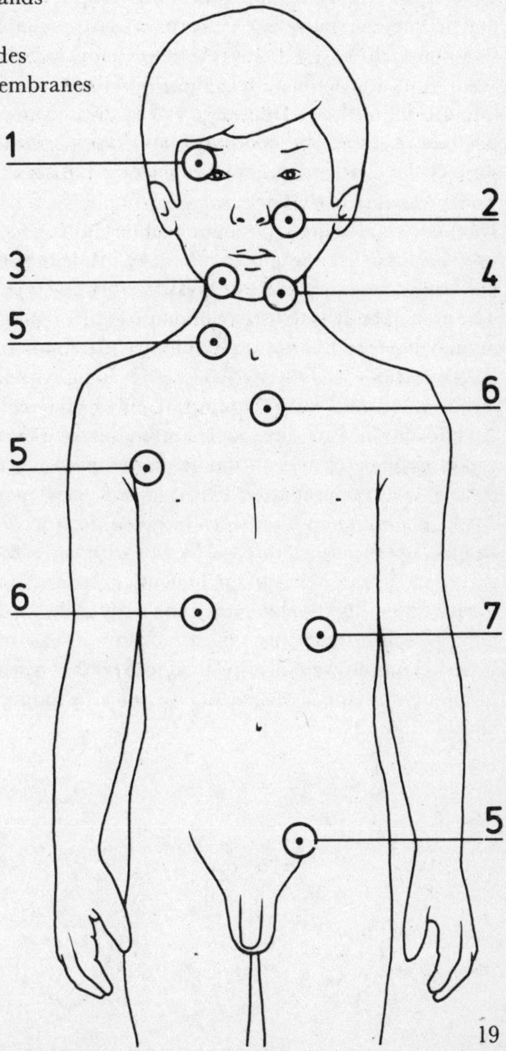

1

2

3

4

5

6

5

6

7

5

immunity

Immunity is the body's natural or induced ability to withstand invasion by disease organisms. The chief source of immunity is the lymphatic system, which includes the spleen and lymph nodes. These manufacture antibodies – large, complex protein molecules that play a major role in the fight against infection. Antibodies attack the protein sheaths of bacteria and viruses by interlocking with and thus inactivating them. In most cases, one type of antibody reacts only to one type of germ. Someone protected by antibodies against a particular disease is said to have immunity to that disease.

Immunity is also brought about by interferons – special proteins that curb the spread of viruses inside the body. Unlike antibodies, interferons are not restricted to one type of target. The human body is naturally immune to many plant and animal diseases. But natural immunity to human disease largely varies with inherited differences in individuals' antibody output. Natural immunity may be passive or active. An unborn child acquires some antibodies from his mother, and after birth receives antibodies in her milk. The result is a passive, natural immunity. This lasts only a few months. Artificial passive immunity can be given to protect instantly against an established disease. Serum with antibodies against the disease is injected into the patient's bloodstream.

Active immunity develops when the body makes antibodies to fight invading organisms. One attack by a disease may produce lifelong immunity against fresh attacks by that disease. Active immunity to some diseases can be artificially induced by vaccination.

vaccination

Vaccines are the most important source of artificial immunity.
They work by exploiting the same natural process in which the
body develops natural immunity against disease organisms
that get in by chance.

Hostile substances in a vaccine provoke the body to make
antibodies against them. Each vaccine gives protection against
a specific disease. Some vaccines give lifelong protection; others
are effective only for months or years.

Vaccines may be made in various ways, employing:

a) dead or inactivated disease organisms (eg influenza
vaccine);

b) weakened live organisms (eg German measles vaccine);

c) a similar organism (eg cowpox virus for smallpox
immunity);

d) toxoids – substances that cause the body to make antitoxins
against poisons produced by disease organisms (eg diphtheria).

why vaccinate?

Vaccination can protect children against many once-common
killing and disabling diseases. Vaccination against smallpox,
tuberculosis, and diphtheria alone has saved millions of lives.
But the resulting decline in such diseases has persuaded many
parents that vaccination is unnecessary. Others, worried by
suggested links between whooping cough vaccine and
encephalitis, think vaccination risky. In fact the risk of death or
bodily damage from whooping cough far outweighs that from
vaccination.

If the proportion of unvaccinated children rises, the risk of
grave epidemic disease among them increases too. So unless
your doctor advises otherwise, accept all the routine childhood
vaccinations.

routine immunization

Described here are all the immunizations normally offered to children in the United Kingdom. This information is intended only as a very general guide to parents. Recommendations vary slightly from area to area, and modifications may be required for some children. Advice can be obtained from the local health clinic or family doctor.

Diphtheria, whooping cough (pertussis), tetanus
Protection against these diseases can be obtained from a combination vaccine (DPT). Alternatively, parents may request that their child be vaccinated only against diphtheria and tetanus. The usual course consists of three DPT injections given at intervals during the child's first year, followed by a booster vaccination against diphtheria and tetanus when the child starts school.

Poliomyelitis Vaccination against polio is usually given at the same time as the DPT injections (including a booster on school entry). The usual polio vaccine is given orally on a sugar lump.

Measles Vaccination against mealses requires a single injection. This is usually given in the second year of life.

German measles (rubella) Vaccination in the form of a single injection is available to girls aged 11–13 years. It is given even to children who have had German measles.

Tuberculosis A test for immunity is usual between 11 and 13 years. Children whose test is positive are referred for X-ray to ensure that they are not suffering from the disease. Children whose test is negative are given a single BCG vaccination. BCG vaccination may be recommended at birth for children with a high risk of contracting the disease (eg, for children in some immigrant families).

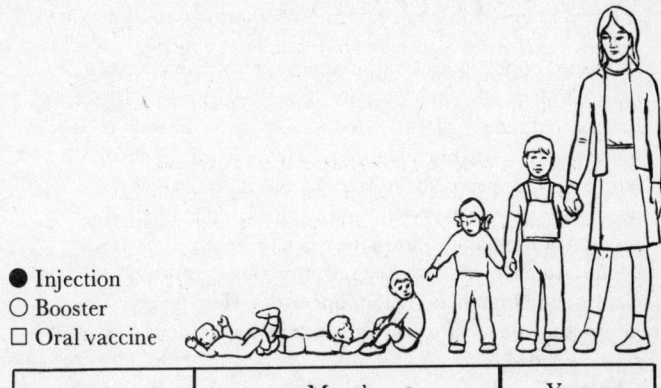

- ● Injection
- ○ Booster
- □ Oral vaccine

	Months				Years	
	3	4½–5	8½–11	12–24	4–5	11–13
Diphtheria	●	●	●		○	
Whooping cough	●	●	●			
Tetanus	●	●	●		○	
Poliomyelitis	□	□	□		□	
Measles				●		
German measles						●
Tuberculosis						●

immunization for foreign travel

Increased opportunities for foreign travel mean that many more children, like their parents, now face the possibility of contracting serious diseases that almost never occur in their home country. Anyone planning a trip to countries outside Northern Europe or North America is advised to seek up-to-date information on required or recommended immunizations. This information can be obtained from your doctor, from foreign embassies, from airline immunization centres, and from holiday tour operators. Here we give information on some of the immunizations that might be recommended.

Cholera This disease is caused by bacteria spread in the faeces of infected people. It is mainly found in countries with inadequate sanitation. Where medical treatment is also inadequate, cholera can kill through dehydration caused by severe vomiting and diarrhoea. A single injection gives some protection for up to six months.

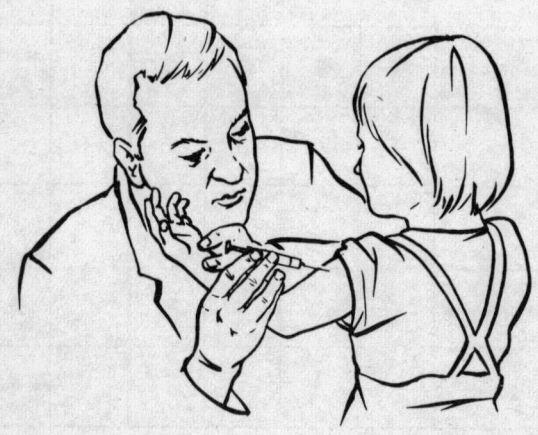

Typhoid Caused by bacteria transmitted in contaminated food and water, typhoid and paratyphoid are common in poorer countries. Potentially fatal complications include intestinal haemorrhage and perforation. A course of two injections gives protection for about two years. Immunity can then be extended by single booster shots every two to three years.

Yellow fever Caused by a virus and spread by mosquito bites, yellow fever occurs in parts of Africa and South America. It affects the liver and kidneys and causes severe jaundice. Fear that the disease will spread to Asia means that travellers to many countries in that continent are required to produce a current vaccination certificate. Vaccination gives immunity for 10 years.

Malaria This tropical disease, caused by a microscopic parasite, is transmitted by mosquito bites. Acute symptoms are chills and high fever. Repeated attacks produce anaemia and enlargement of the liver and spleen. As yet there is no vaccination for malaria, but protection can be obtained by taking preventive tablets before, during, and for one month after a visit to countries where malaria is prevalent.

medical treatment of infection

The body's defences do not easily subdue all infections, but many can be crushed by antibiotics and sulphonamide drugs. Antibiotics are chemicals made by microorganisms. They halt the growth of or kill bacteria, fungi, and rickettsias by interfering with nutrient absorption and cell formation. Some act against only a small group of microbes: others (broad spectrum antibiotics) attack a wide range of targets. Antibiotics have no effect on viral infections.

Diseases susceptible to antibiotics include dysentery, scarlet fever or strep rash, tuberculosis, typhoid, and many minor infections.

Sulphonamides (or sulpha drugs) are synthetic chemicals all of which contain the elements sulphur, hydrogen, nitrogen, and oxygen. They work by blocking the production of certain chemicals that bacteria need in order to grow.

Some sulpha drugs are used against general infection of the body, others for local action in the intestinal tract and for certain bladder infections.

Sulpha drugs have proved useful against blood poisoning, dysentery, meningitis, pneumonia, and some other diseases. But for most purposes, antibiotics have replaced sulpha drugs. Neither attacks viruses and some bacteria have evolved resistance to antibiotics.

common early rashes

Rashes are common skin conditions in the first few months of life. These rashes are usually insignificant and reflect the reaction of the young baby's skin to external conditions. Treatment may be needed, however, if the rash looks infected.

Prickly heat appears on the neck and shoulders of babies in hot weather, and may spread to the chest, arms, and face. It forms a rash of pink pimples surrounded by blotches of pink skin. The pimples may blister. It is usually caused by dressing the baby too warmly.

Mild face rash may occur as tiny white pimples, small red pimples that take longer to go away, or rough red patches. The cause is unknown. Such rashes will clear up in time without treatment.

Nappy rash occurs as patches of redness and spots in the nappy area and is a cause of great discomfort. It can result from sensitivity to soap, bleaches, or fabric rinses used on the nappies, from powders or lotions applied to the skin, from yeast infections, or from irritation caused by wet or dirty nappies. In older babies it is often caused by the reaction of the skin to ammonia formed by the interaction of stools with urea in the urine. To treat the condition: boil the nappies for at least 10 minutes and rinse with an antiseptic rinse, use one-way liners or disposable nappies, change towelling nappies as often as possible, and do not use waterproof pants. Use a cream on the nappy area and expose the area to the air as much as possible.

skin conditions

Eczema is an allergic skin condition in which patches of rough, red, scaly skin cause intense irritation. It is most common in children with a family history of eczema or other allergic conditions such as hay fever or asthma. Causes include foods, and external irritants such as soap or wool. It may be aggravated by nervous tension. In a young baby, eczema most often begins on the cheeks or forehead. Later, it may occur anywhere on the body, especially in the elbow creases and behind the knees. The condition may improve or disappear as the child gets older. Cortisone ointment may be prescribed in severe cases, but should not be over-used. Emulsifying ointments can provide significant relief.

Hives, or nettle rash, is another form of allergic skin reaction. Characterized by painful, itchy skin weals, it may be caused by certain types of food, drug, or insect bite. Hives may also result from emotional tension. The condition is not normally serious, and soothing lotions will ease the child's discomfort. Medical attention must, however, be sought if swellings that may affect breathing occur in the area of the mouth and throat.

Chilblains are itching, red swellings that occur on the extremities as a result of poor circulation in cold weather. Scratching may lead to infection. Warm clothing is the best form of protection.

Treatment may be with drugs, or by improving circulation through exercise.

Swollen red hands may occur in babies in cold weather. The condition disappears once the baby is warm again. Avoid the problem by ensuring that the baby's hands are always well protected from cold.

Cradle cap This is a very common condition in young babies. A yellowish, waxy crust or dry scales form on the baby's scalp, and it is important that these should be removed to avoid the risk of infection. Massaging the baby's scalp with baby oil before normal washing will help loosen the scales.

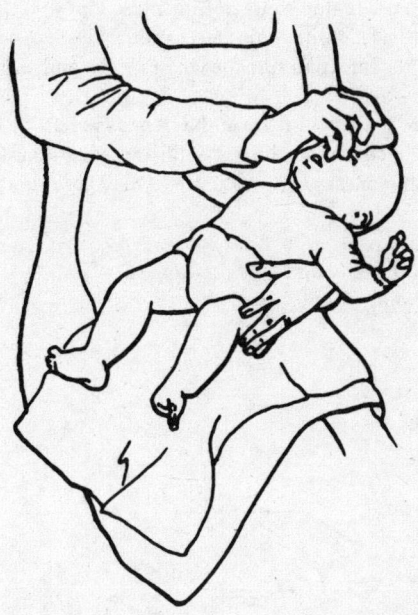

skin infections

Ringworm is a very contagious fungus infection affecting the skin and sometimes the nails. Scaly, crusted lumps form circular patches that clear in the centre and spread out from the site of the infection. On the scalp, ringworm often causes the hair to break off short. Ringworm can now be effectively treated with drugs.

Athlete's foot is caused by a fungus that thrives in wet, warm conditions. The skin between the toes becomes white, soft, wet, and itchy. The condition is made worse by perspiration. Good general foot care is essential, and fungicide ointments should be used.

Impetigo is a highly contagious bacterial infection. It usually starts on the face with a pimple that develops into a brown crusty scab. Impetigo spreads very rapidly, and antibiotics may be needed.

Cold sore is a virus infection that tends to recur. A stinging sensation gives rise to clusters of blisters that dry up in about 10 days. Commonest near the mouth, it may occur in the genital area.

Ringworm
1 Scaly, crusted lumps
2 Epidermis
3 Dermis

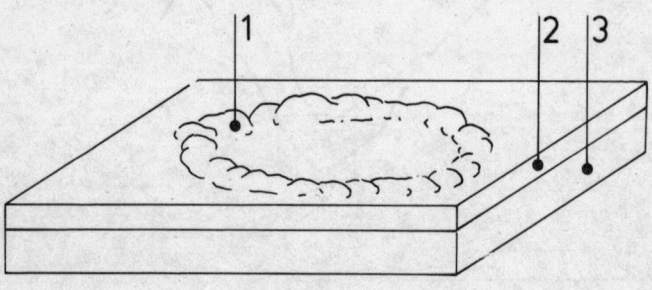

Warts are small harmless growths caused by a virus. Some will disappear without treatment, or they can be treated at home with chemical applications or surgically removed by a doctor. Always seek medical advice about warts on the feet (verrucas).

Boils are painful, pus-filled lumps caused by bacterial infection of a hair follicle, a sebaceous or sweat gland, or a break in the skin. They are most common where the skin is rubbed by clothing, and usually burst after several days. Most need only a protective dressing, but a doctor should be consulted if the child is very young or if several boils occur.

Acne is an infective skin condition common in adolescence. The oil-producing sebaceous glands become clogged and infected resulting in pimples, blackheads, whiteheads, and sometimes boils and cysts. Face, neck, shoulders, chest, and back are often affected. Most cases of acne clear up in time but attention should be paid to hygiene and choice of cosmetics. Treatments include lotions and creams. Antibiotics may be needed in severe cases.

Boil

1 Pus-filled cavity
2 Core
3 Dead tissue

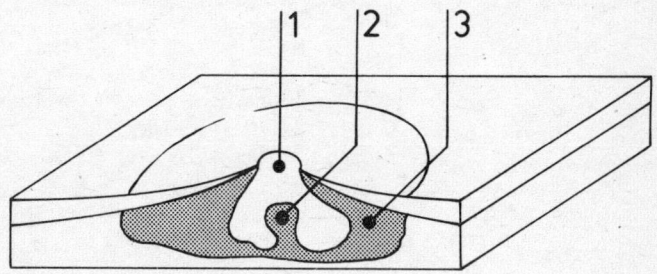

disease rashes

Many rashes in childhood are insignificant, but others are signs of infectious diseases. To avoid mistakes in identification the doctor should always be consulted if a child with a rash appears in any other way unwell (also see pp. 44–47).

1 Measles rash develops on the third to the fifth day of the illness, after which the child usually begins to feel better. The rash is of dark red spots that merge into blotches. It usually begins behind the ears and then spreads over the body.

2 German measles produces a light pink rash that begins on the neck and face and gradually spreads over the body. Often the spots merge to give a flushed appearance. The rash is often the first sign of illness and lasts only a few days.

3 Chicken pox rash is often the first sign of illness. Commonest on face, scalp, and chest, and sometimes found in the mouth, spots appear over a three-day period. The rash consists of dark red pimples on which blisters develop a few hours after appearance. These burst easily and scabs form. Unless they are scratched – when permanent scars may result – the scabs fall off to leave pink scars that soon fade. Calamine lotion reduces itching.

4 Scarlet fever or strep rash appears on the second day, spreading over the body from damp areas such as the groin, armpits, and sometimes the back. The rash is made up of tiny red spots on a flushed skin. The area around the mouth remains white. After a week, the skin over the spots begins to peel.

1 Measles
2 German measles
3 Chicken pox
4 Scarlet fever

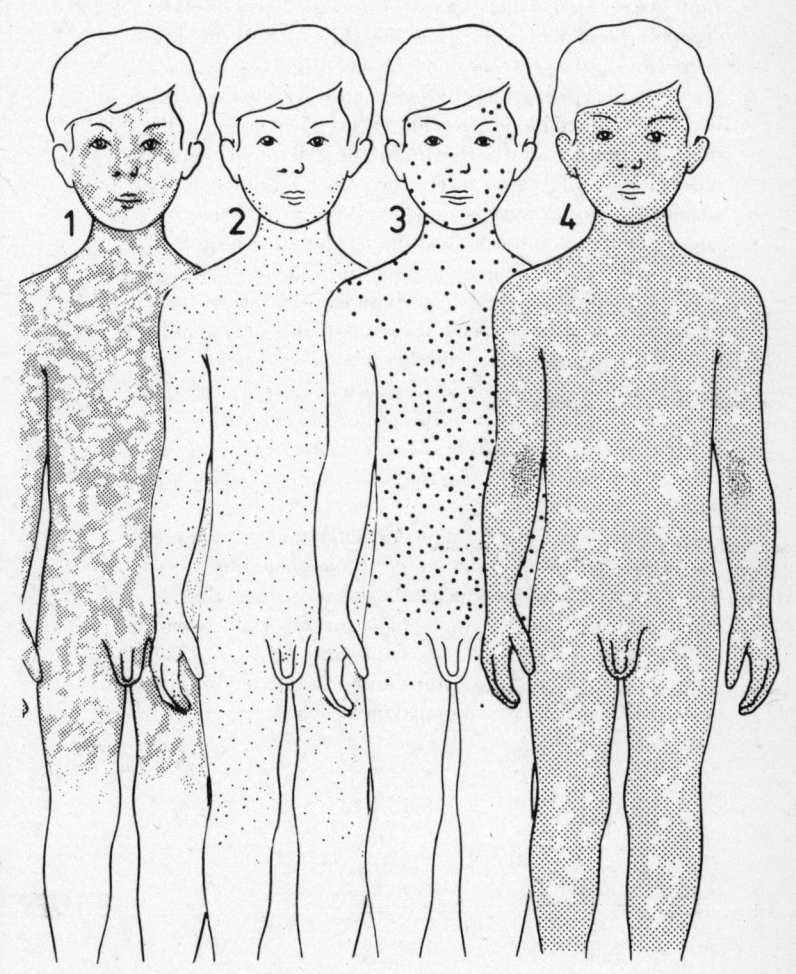

jaundice

Jaundice is a sign of disorder rather than an illness itself. In jaundice the skin and sometimes the whites of the eyes appear yellow due to the presence in the blood of an excess of bile pigment. This pigment is produced in the liver by the normal breakdown of red blood cells. The excess bile pigment in the blood in jaundice may be due to a number of causes, requiring different types of treatment. For this reason it is important to consult a doctor as soon as jaundice is suspected. Other signs of jaundice are dark urine and pale faeces. Jaundice is quite common in newborn babies, among which the most usual cause is simple inefficiency of the liver. Jaundice of this type usually disappears after a few days, but special treatment is sometimes needed. In very rare cases jaundice in a baby is due to congenital defect: the baby is born with no duct to carry bile away from the liver. An important cause of jaundice in newborn infants results from rhesus incompatibility between mother and baby; preventive treatment is now available to mothers whose babies are at risk.

Rare in infants but more common in older children is jaundice due to infection. Most common is infectious hepatitis, transmitted by food or drink handled by a carrier of the hepatitis virus. It may occur in epidemics, especially where hygiene is poor. Preventive vaccination may be given. Less common is serum hepatitis, transmitted by infected blood used in transfusion or by contaminated medical instruments.

1 Liver
2 Gall bladder
3 Bile duct
4 Duodenum

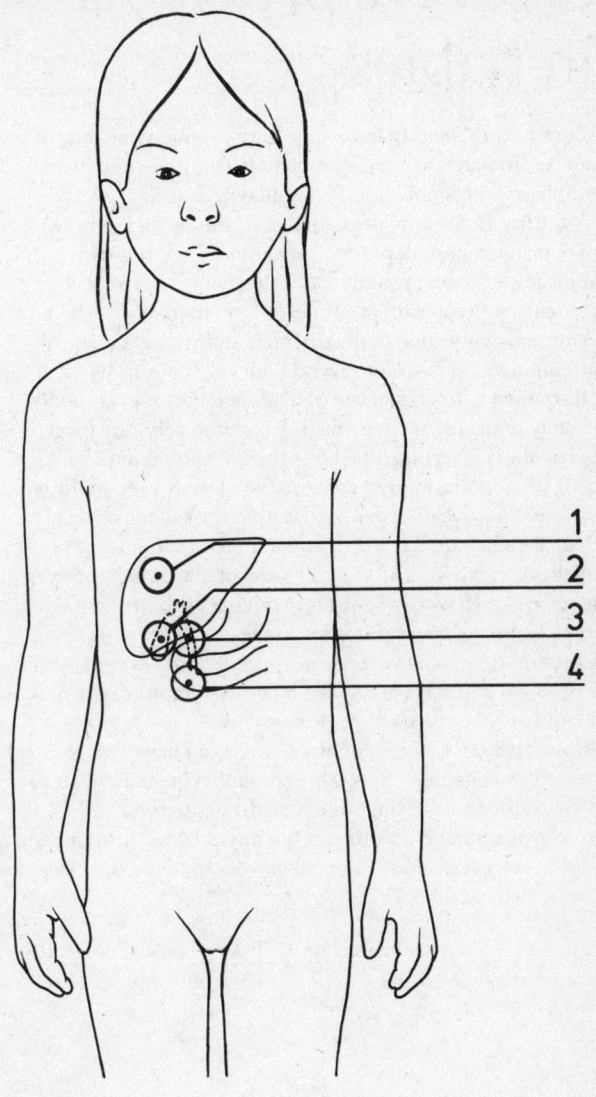

1
2
3
4

digestive problems in babies

Digestive problems in babies are very common and may or may not be serious. Warning signs include vomiting, diarrhoea, problems with stools, and abdominal pain.

Vomiting in the form of gentle regurgitation, or 'spitting' of milk is quite normal, particularly after a feed. But true vomiting – the regurgitation and ejection of the stomach's contents with some force – is much less common. It may be a symptom of infection or obstruction, and requires medical attention if it persists for several hours or contains blood or bile.

Diarrhoea in infants, particularly when the onset is sudden, usually indicates an intestinal infection; in very rare cases, particularly if accompanied by other symptoms such as coughing or intermittent constipation, it may even indicate a serious digestive disorder. Either way, the sudden onset of diarrhoea in babies is a serious complaint that must have medical attention. The gradual onset of diarrhoea, however, may be caused by carelessness in mixing feeds or the introduction of new substances to the diet.

Constipation occurs mainly in bottle-fed babies, and is rarely a problem unless accompanied by other symptoms. Laxatives should only be given on medical advice.

Blood in stools Streaks of blood can result from fissure in anus caused by constipation. A large amount of blood indicates a serious disorder needing urgent medical attention.

Stools of unusual colour can be caused by the introduction of new foods, overconcentration of powder in the feed, or from the use of medicinal iron.

Abdominal pain during a baby's early months may well indicate colic. This is a severe abdominal pain that affects many babies between the ages of two weeks and three months. Attacks usually occur daily, often in the evening, and can last up to four hours. Typically a baby with colic refuses to settle down after the late afternoon or early evening feed, begins to scream and draws his legs up sharply. The baby can be comforted temporarily if cuddled or wrapped up tightly, but distress returns as soon as he is left again. The causes of colic are uncertain and medical opinion is still in disagreement. Some doctors, however, suggest some precautions that may possibly prevent an attack. The baby should not be allowed to feed too quickly; he should be thoroughly burped after a feed; and he should be kept warm.

Milk allergy A very few babies who fail to thrive are found to be allergic to milk. This allergy is identified by a series of hospital tests, after which the doctor will prescribe the use of a special non-milk formula. A baby fed on a special non-milk formula can be expected to have normal rates of growth.

digestive problems in older children

Digestive problems in children have many causes. Signs include vomiting (see p. 63), stomachache, diarrhoea, and constipation.

In general, the doctor should be consulted if the parent is at all worried by the child's condition, particularly if warning signs occur together, if the child has a fever, or if abdominal pain is at all persistent.

Stomachache Many young children complain of a stomachache when they really mean that they feel unwell; perhaps if they are about to vomit. Other children develop a quite genuine stomachache when they are tense or worried. A common cause of stomachache in children is the onset of another illness such as a cold, throat infection, or influenza. Other causes are appendicitis (see p. 39) and intestinal infections that also cause sickness and diarrhoea.

Diarrhoea is seldom significant in itself, although it may be an early indication of a more serious ailment. If diarrhoea occurs with vomiting there is a danger of dehydration if the condition persists. The doctor should be called at once to a child of any age who is unable to take fluids.

Constipation may sometimes be a sign of illness – if the child is eating or drinking less, or if fluid has been lost through fever or vomiting. One problem, usually a passing phase, is that young children 'hold back' their bowel movements until they are hard and difficult to pass. More usually, however, constipation is a condition imagined by parents.

appendicitis

The appendix is a small closed tube leading off the large intestine. In appendicitis it becomes inflamed, usually as a result of a blockage. Sometimes the condition develops very rapidly, becoming critical in 24 hours or so. Often the first symptom is pain around the navel, which then changes to a pain in the right of the abdomen. Tenderness in the area over the appendix – McBurney's point – is a distinctive feature. Nausea is common, and vomiting and fever may occur.

It is important to call a doctor at once if appendicitis is suspected; without prompt medical attention the appendix may burst, causing peritonitis which can be fatal. Do not give laxatives or treat for indigestion. Cases of acute appendicitis are treated by prompt surgical removal of the appendix.

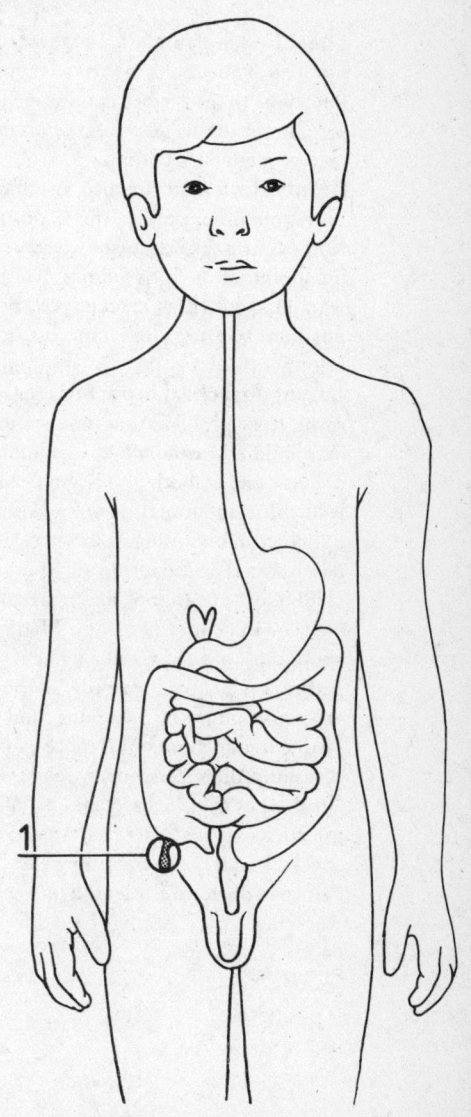

1 Appendix

respiratory problems

Tonsillitis, inflammation of the tonsils, is a symptom of a number of infectious diseases ranging from minor throat infections to the serious condition known as strep throat. Any sore throat that is persistent or accompanied by fever should receive medical attention.

Bronchitis is acute or chronic inflammation of the bronchial tubes, but other parts of the respiratory tract are also affected. Mucus gathers and causes wheezy breathing and coughing. Sometimes bronchitis follows a cold, influenza, measles, whooping cough, or chicken pox. Bronchitis may itself lead to pneumonia. Drugs, inhalations, and physiotherapy are used in treatment.

Laryngo-tracheal bronchitis (croup) This is a very serious respiratory problem that requires urgent medical attention. The child has usually had a common cold, perhaps followed by a severe and sometimes violent cough. In laryngo-tracheal bronchitis inflammation of the larynx and trachea results in difficulty in breathing, sometimes associated with a loud, harsh sound as the respiratory passages become blocked. The child may appear grey, and increasing restlessness indicates the onset of an acute emergency. Medical help should be summoned at the first suspicion of this condition.

Asthma is a chronic disorder of the bronchial tubes causing attacks of wheezing, coughing, and difficult breathing. It may be due to infection, but is more usually an inherited allergic reaction. Allergic asthma is made worse by emotional stress. Antibiotics may be used against infection, and desensitizing injections against allergies. An attack may be controlled with a special inhaler, and breathing exercises may be useful. Always call your doctor if the length or severity of an attack is worrying.

Pneumonia is acute inflammation of the lungs. Symptoms include fever, chest pains, and a harsh, dry cough. The infection may be patchy, usually around the bronchial tubes (bronchopneumonia), or may affect an entire lung (lobar pneumonia). When body resistance is low, pneumonia may be caused by bacteria usually present in the mouth and throat. Bronchopneumonia is often a complication of another illness, or may be caused by foreign matter such as food in the lungs. Treatment is with antibiotics or sulphonamide drugs.

1 Tonsillitis
2 Laryngo-tracheal bronchitis
3 Bronchitis
4 Asthma
5 Pneumonia

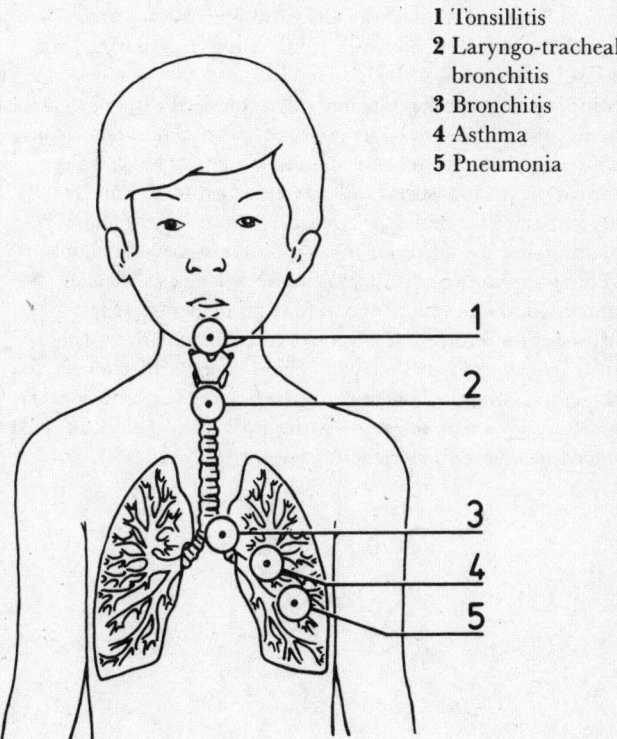

ear problems

Earache is common in children and should always be taken seriously. A doctor should be consulted at once whenever a child suffers from earache, discharge from the ear, or deafness.

Outer-ear problems are commonly due to infection or allergy. Typical causes of infection are the presence of a foreign body in the ear, and scratching the ear with unclean fingers. Allergic reactions, sometimes leading to secondary infection, may result from chemicals, metals, and topical use of antibiotics. Symptoms include itching, redness in the ear canal, and often pain and a discharge, with temporary deafness if the discharge blocks the canal. Wipe away any surplus discharge, and consult a doctor. Do not wash out the ear as this may help spread infection.

Middle-ear infection is commonly associated with infections of the nose and throat, and may be of bacterial or viral origin. The symptoms may include an initial feeling of blockage in the ear, which increases to a deep-seated earache. This is accompanied by toxicity and fever. Hearing may be affected, and the severity of hearing loss will increase with the build-up of discharge in the ear. Always consult a doctor at once: if untreated, the condition may lead to permanent deafness.

Mastoiditis Middle-ear infections can spread to the mastoid bone – the part of the skull just behind the ear. Infection swells the skin around the bone, causing pain and fever. Treatment is with antibiotics. In severe cases surgical removal of the infected bone (mastoidectomy) may be necessary.

Deafness can be temporary or permanent, caused by obstructions or disease. Congenital deafness can be due to genetic defect or to infections (eg German measles) during the mother's pregnancy. If deafness is suspected in a baby, specialist help should be sought at once. Warning signs of deafness in a baby are that he continues to 'babble' long after others are using recognizable words.

1 Ear canal
2 Ear drum
3 Middle ear
4 Eustachian tube
5 Mastoid bone

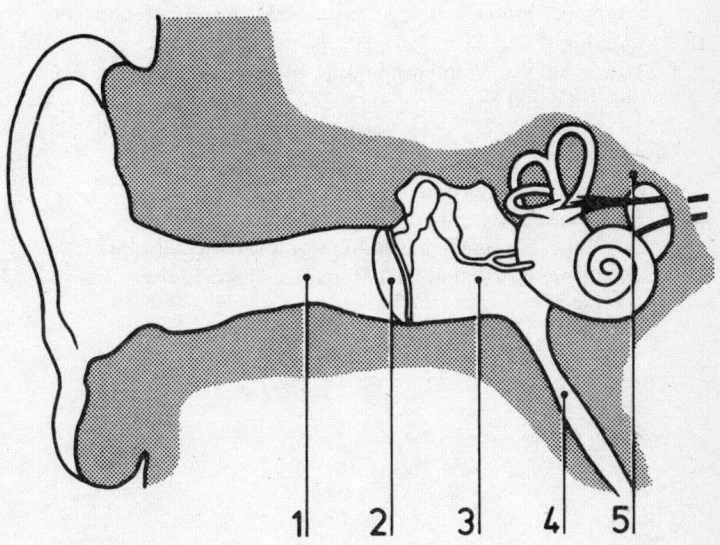

infectious diseases

Bacterial meningitis
Incubation: 1–10 days.
Symptoms: In young babies: lassitude, irritability, poor feeding, convulsions, fever, vomiting, possible increase in head size. In older children: headache, fever, vomiting, convulsions, neck rigidity, rash.
Treatment: Immediate antibiotics.

Chicken pox
Incubation: 12–21 days.
Symptoms: Chill, fever, headache, malaise. Red spots – on face, chest, back – that later contain clear fluid, burst, and develop brown crusts.
Treatment: For symptoms only: rest, and lotion for itching.

Coughs and colds
Incubation: 12–36 hours.
Symptoms: Stuffy or runny nose, raised temperature, possibly vomiting.
Treatment: For symptoms: liquids, paracetamol to reduce fever (see p. 62) and rest.

Diphtheria
Incubation: 2–5 days.
Symptoms: Fever, sore throat, swollen neck glands, may be a dark, offensive-smelling membrane at the back of the throat.
Treatment: Heavy doses of antitoxin, and sometimes antibiotics.

Gastroenteritis
Incubation: 0–24 hours.
Symptoms: Continual vomiting, diarrhoea, irritability,
dehydration.
Treatment: In babies, reduce feeding of milk and any solids,
and give clear liquids, eg dextrose in boiled water.

German measles (Rubella)
Incubation: 14–21 days.
Symptoms: Malaise, headache, inflamed mucous membrane,
in rare cases fever. Fine pink spots first on face and neck, and
then elsewhere.
Treatment: For symptoms: lotion for itching, paracetamol or
similar analgesic (see p. 62) for headache.

Measles
Incubation: 10–14 days.
Symptoms: Fever, cough, conjunctivitis (red eyes). Allover rash
appears later – white spots with red perimeter, along with
inflamed background skin.
Treatment: For symptoms: rest, cough syrup, soft diet,
protection from cold, damp, and bright light. Treatment also
for any complications.

Infectious mononucleosis (Glandular fever)
Incubation: Approximately 1 week.
Symptoms: Headache, fever, sore throat, swollen lymph nodes,
loss of appetite.
Treatment: For symptoms: rest, mouthwash, an analgesic (see
p. 62). Treatment for complications, if any.

infectious diseases continued

Mumps
Incubation: 14–28 days.
Symptoms: Chill and fever, headache, temperature, swollen salivary glands (pain on chewing). Other glands may be swollen.
Treatment: For symptoms: rest, soft diet, an analgesic (see p. 62), perhaps a sedative.
In the United Kingdom it is unusual to be immunized against mumps.

Poliomyelitis (Polio)
Incubation: 7–14 days.
Symptoms: Minor: fever, headache, diarrhoea, vomiting (this stage lasts 1–2 days). Major (beginning 7 days later): fever, stiff neck, tender muscles, severe restlessness. May go on to paralytic stage: weak muscles, asymmetrical paralysis possibly affecting breathing. Improves after 7 days but may leave residual disability.
Treatment: Bed rest and sedatives. In paralytic stage, massage of affected muscles and possibly use of a respirator.

Rheumatic fever
Incubation: 1–6 weeks.
Symptoms: Sore throat, fever, diffuse rash, pains in limbs and large joints, may be small rheumatic nodules beneath the skin.
Treatment: Bed rest, an analgesic (see p. 62), prolonged use of penicillin in large doses, and occasionally steroid hormones.

Roseola
Incubation: 4–7 days.
Symptoms: May be convulsions at onset. High fever 3–4 days.
Purple-brown spots on chest, abdomen, face, and extremities.
Treatment: For symptoms only: an analgesic (see p. 62), water
sponging to lower temperature.

Scarlet fever or Strep rash
Incubation: 1–3 days.
Symptoms: Chills, fever, vomiting. Rash 24 hours after fever:
small red spots join to form redness on whole body. Strawberry
tongue. Sore throat.
Treatment: Penicillin, rest, soft diet, water sponging to lower
temperature, lotions for itching.

Viral meningitis; Encephalitis
Incubation: 0–7 days.
Symptoms: As for bacterial meningitis.
Treatment: Supportive treatment. Antibiotics to prevent
recurrence.

Whooping cough
Incubation: 7–14 days.
Symptoms: Sneezing, listlessness, and cough becoming
convulsive with typical whooping breathing. Vomiting. May
expel thick mucus.
Treatment: Rest, fresh air, small meals, refeeding after
vomiting. Mild sedatives and antibiotics. Hospital for serious
cases.

fleas, lice, and mites

Infestation by various parasites is common among children. Some types of parasite live by biting the skin of animals and humans to suck their blood. They cause irritation and may spread disease.

Fleas The flea that usually lives on man (Pulex irritans) causes severe irritation. Some animal fleas also bite man – most serious are the bites of the rat flea, which spread typhus and bubonic plague. Eggs are laid in floorboard cracks, in beds, and on pets. Fleas are best controlled by strict cleanliness.

Body lice live and lay their eggs in the seams of clothing. Infested clothing should be washed and sterilized in boiling water. Body lice spread typhus, and bites may be sources of other infection.

Head lice live on the scalp, laying tiny, white, sticky eggs (nits) on the hair. It is easiest to detect head lice by finding the eggs. There may also be itching red spots where the hair meets the back of the neck. Head lice are not known to spread disease. but bites may become sites of infection. The scalp should be treated several times with specially formulated lotion or shampoo, and the hair combed with a fine-toothed comb. Insecticides should not be used.

Mites Bites by the itch mite cause scabies – groups of scabbed pimples frequently occurring on the backs of the hands, the wrists, penis, and stomach. Scabies is contagious and requires medical treatment. The usual remedy is benzylbenzoate, painted on the skin. Chiggers, or harvest mites, are found in some countries and cause itching, blotching, and blisters. They can be removed with soap and water.

(See p. 50 for illustrations.)

parasitic worms

Several types of parasitic worm can live in the intestines of humans.

Threadworms, or pinworms, are fairly common in children. About ¼in (6mm) long, they resemble tiny white threads. They live in the intestine but come out at night to lay their eggs around the anus, where they cause itching. Mild stomach pains, nausea and diarrhoea may also occur, and worms can be seen in the faeces. Eggs are spread on sheets and hands. Treatment is easy, but first consult a doctor.

Common roundworms invade intestines, liver, and lungs. They are up to 4in (10cm) long and look like earthworms. There may be no symptoms unless a great many worms are present, in which case an obstruction of the bile duct may occur. Microscopic eggs are passed in the faeces, and are spread in contaminated food. A doctor will prescribe effective treatment.

Tapeworms Several types of tapeworm are found in man, usually caught from inadequately cooked beef, fish, or pork. Tapeworms may grow 30ft (9m) long, and attach themselves to the intestinal wall by suckers or hooks on the head. Body segments break off and are passed in the faeces. Only the larva of the pork tapeworm develops in man. Effective drugs are available.

Hookworms Commonest in tropical countries, hookworms are about ½in (1.27cm) long and attach themselves to the intestine wall to suck blood. Symptoms are unusual appetite, constipation alternating with diarrhoea, anaemia, and malnutrition. Eggs are passed out in the faeces. Larvae enter the body by burrowing into bare feet. Treatment is by drugs, high-protein diet, and iron supplements.

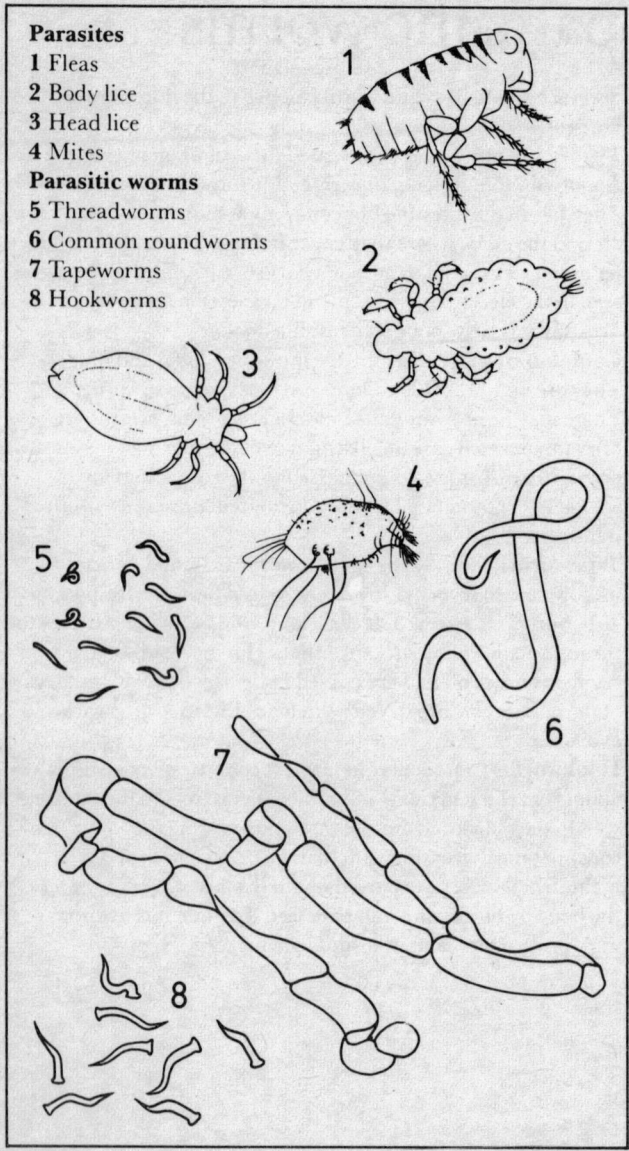

Parasites
1 Fleas
2 Body lice
3 Head lice
4 Mites
Parasitic worms
5 Threadworms
6 Common roundworms
7 Tapeworms
8 Hookworms

infantile convulsions

Some young children are prone to infantile convulsions, also called febrile convulsions. They are usually brought on by high fever and are best avoided by keeping fever down (see p. 62). A convulsion lasts at most for a few minutes, but may be alarming. The child loses consciousness, and starts to twitch and shake. His eyes roll, his teeth are clenched, his breathing is heavy, and he may froth at the mouth or wet himself. A convulsion always ends in sleep. The child must not be left alone until the convulsion ends, because of the risk of inhaling vomit (his head should be turned to one side if he vomits). His limbs should be kept away from danger but no attempt made to restrain him or to hold down his tongue. The doctor should be called after the child has gone to sleep.

epilepsy

Occasionally convulsions in infants may be a sign of epilepsy, a disorder of the nervous system that may be due to brain damage but may also be inherited. There are two main types of epilepsy: petit mal and grand mal. Both can be controlled by drugs.

Petit mal is characterized by momentary lapses of attention, sometimes with blinking or slight twitching. Attacks last only a few seconds, but may occur several times in a day. In many cases the sufferer is unaware that anything has happened.

Grand mal is a more severe form of epilepsy in which actual fits occur: the sufferer loses consciousness and has convulsions in which he thrashes about and may foam at the mouth. A fit usually lasts from one to five minutes, and is often followed by sleep (see p. 95 for first aid).

hernias

A hernia occurs when an organ protrudes through a weak point in the muscle around it. Two types of hernia are common in children and may affect both boys and girls.

Umbilical hernia, visible as puffing out of the navel when the child cries, occurs when a small portion of the intestine protrudes through a gap in the abdominal wall left by the umbilical vessels. An umbilical hernia rarely causes trouble, and the gap usually closes after a few weeks or months. Surgery may be recommended if the hernia is still present when the child is two.

Inguinal hernia is potentially more serious and is usually corrected by simple surgery soon after it is discovered, often in the first year. It is most common in boys, occurring when part of the intestine is pushed during crying or straining through the inguinal canal into the groin or scrotum. In girls, inguinal hernia produces a swelling in the groin. Occasionally an inguinal hernia becomes strangulated – trapped so that its blood supply is cut off, causing pain and vomiting. Immediate surgery is required in such cases because of the risk of gangrene or peritonitis.

1 Umbilical hernia
2 Inguinal hernia

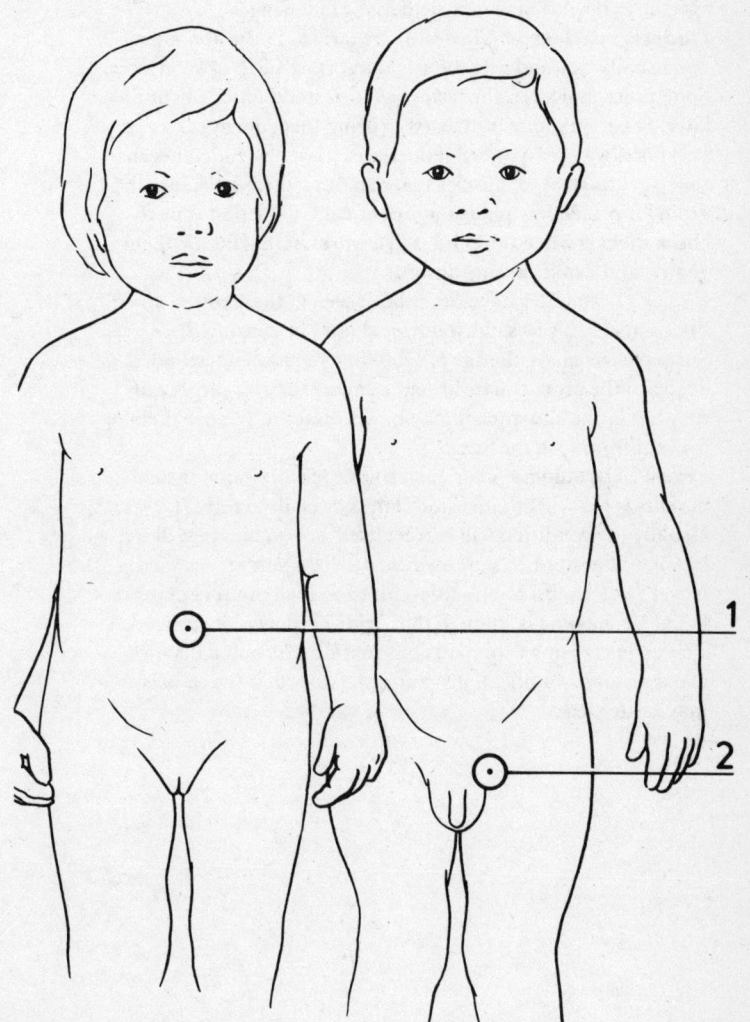

1

2

genital problems

Other problems that may occur include genital problems specific to boys. These can include the following.

Undescended testes The testes are formed in the abdomen and usually descend into the scrotum before birth or soon after. Sometimes, however, the testes fail to descend naturally until later, or surgery may be needed to bring them down.

It is not always easy to tell if the testes have descended because they are attached to muscles that can draw them back into the groin for protection against injury or cold. (The best time to check them is when the child is in a warm bath. Handle them gently, and avoid causing alarm.)

If one or both testes have never been seen in the scrotum when the child is two years old, a doctor should be consulted.

Surgery is usual by the age of six if they remain undescended. Testes in the groin can be brought down easily by surgery; if they are in the abdomen it may be necessary to remove them to prevent trouble in the future.

Foreskin problems A common source of worry among new parents is that their baby's foreskin is difficult to retract. Usually the condition will correct itself as the child gets older, but do not hesitate to seek medical advice if you are worried. Never force back a baby's foreskin. In a small number of cases the penis opening is so small that urine outflow is obstructed. The child screams with pain on urination. Consult a doctor to avoid serious complications. Surgical correction (circumcision) may be needed.

Hypospadias is a congenital deformity of the penis in which the opening of the urethra is on the shaft and not at the tip. It is usually discovered at birth and to ensure normal functioning can be corrected surgically.

Hydrocele In this condition an excess of fluid protecting the testes causes swelling of the scrotum, often on both sides. In babies, the swelling usually disappears without treatment. If it occurs later in life, it may be treated by drawing off some of the fluid, or by surgery.

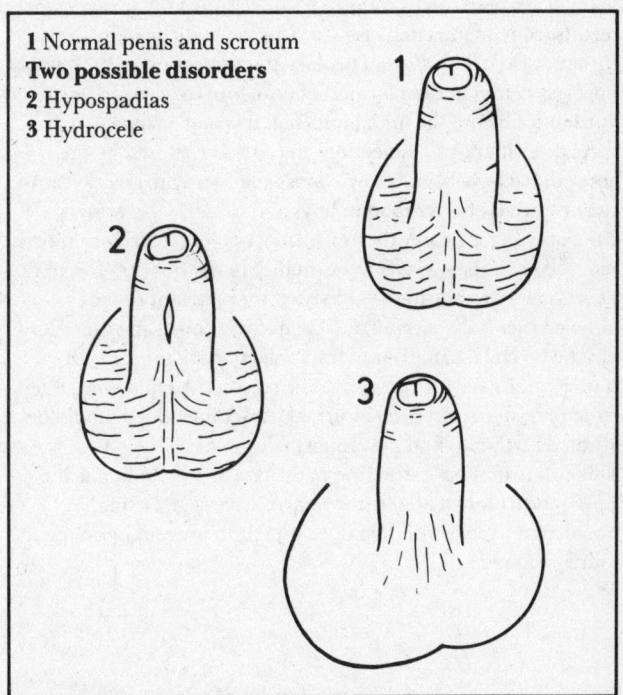

1 Normal penis and scrotum
Two possible disorders
2 Hypospadias
3 Hydrocele

urinary tract problems

Infections may occur anywhere in the urinary tract – kidneys, ureters, bladder, or urethra. They are fairly common in young children, when they may be difficult to diagnose since it is not always apparent that the child is finding urination painful or is urinating abnormally often. Other symptoms – such as vomiting and fever – may have many causes. For this reason a urine test is usual whenever a child has an unexplained fever, or if any fever persists. In some cases infection of the urinary tract results from an infection elsewhere in the body, usually in the throat or ears. This type of urinary tract infection is, however, now less common than formerly because of the use of antibiotics before the initial infection has had a chance to spread. Urinary tract infections may also be caused by the entry of bacteria from below – most commonly in girls because the urethra is shorter than in boys and because the urinary tract opening is nearer the anus. Infection of the urinary tract is more likely if there is any abnormality in the system. To avoid permanent damage to the kidneys it is important that any abnormality is discovered and treated as soon as possible. Any child who has had a urinary tract infection should be kept under careful observation for some months. A child who suffers from persistent or recurrent urinary tract infections should be studied further to find any abnormality.

Difficult urination – straining to urinate or a dribbling urine flow – indicates an abnormally narrow passage or small opening, and requires urgent treatment to prevent permanent kidney damage.

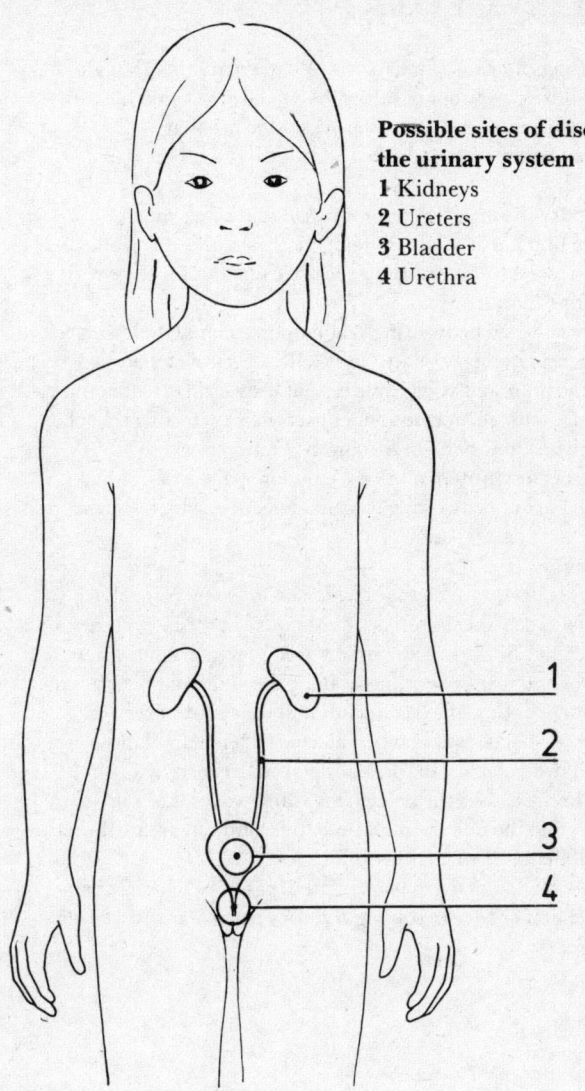

Possible sites of disorder in the urinary system
1 Kidneys
2 Ureters
3 Bladder
4 Urethra

bedwetting

Bedwetting can cause anxiety to child and parents. Though most children grow out of the problem, aids are available to help encourage dryness. In some cases the problem is compounded by soiling the bed.

Causes

Staying dry through the night is a skill that some young children find particularly difficult. In these cases the problem usually results from a small or sensitive bladder together with a large urine output.

In other children bedwetting is a temporary lapse, following a prolonged period of night dryness. Often occurring between the ages of four and seven, this type of bedwetting is often the result of a short-term emotional upset such as starting school or the birth of a new baby in the family. Only very rarely is bedwetting a symptom of severe emotional disturbance. A further cause of bedwetting is urinal infection, which requires prompt medical attention.

Treatment

Here we concentrate on cases where no infection is involved. In general it is sensible to restrict fluid intake in the late afternoon and evening. Because urine production is greatest in the first couple of hours after bedtime, waking the child and taking him to the toilet at this time is often all that is needed to keep his bed dry. A special pad and bell alarm is often helpful in severe cases. A drop of urine on the pad, placed between two undersheets, causes the bell to ring – and wakes the child in time to go to the toilet. An alarm of this kind can greatly boost the confidence of an anxious child.

In rare cases, a doctor may feel that drugs or psychiatric help offer the best chance of solving a child's particular bedwetting problem.

home care

General points

1) Lethargy, loss of appetite, or slight fever indicate the onset of many childhood illnesses.

2) If such a condition develops, put the child to bed; if it worsens, consult a doctor, who may prescribe medicine and advise on diet and overall care.

3) Some illnesses are infectious and require isolation.

4) Sick children may need help with simple, everyday actions.

5) They need solicitude but not pampering.

6) Cheerful patients often recover faster than gloomy ones, so as far as possible keep your sick child occupied.

7) In cases of infectious disease, maintain a scrupulous hygiene. Keep the child's crockery and cutlery separate (or use disposables) and watch any relatives and friends for signs and symptoms.

Increasing comfort

A sick child may easily become lonely, miserable, and bored. Try to make his room bright and attractive. If he is well enough to sit up, build a soft wall of pillows to support his back. Remove crumbs and wrinkles from his sheets. These need changing often, and if bedwetting is a problem, put a rubber sheet below them. A bedside table placed in easy reach should hold favourite books, magazines and games, a radio, and drinking water. If he is strong enough, a short period sitting on a chair or on the bed will help relieve monotony. Be solicitous but practical: resist continual attention seeking, but spend set times with him. In a long illness avoid showing too much concern.

how to take
a temperature

The temperature can be taken in the mouth, rectum, or armpit
(the latter gives a reading approximately 1°F : 0.5°C below the
others). Do not take the temperature soon after the child has
eaten or drunk anything, or had a bath.

First rinse the thermometer in cold water, and wipe it dry.
Place it in the appropriate position (for an oral reading the bulb
should be under the tongue, and the mouth kept closed).
Remove the thermometer after three minutes. Holding the end
opposite the bulb, read the silver column of mercury against
the scale. Make a note of the temperature. Shake down the
mercury column. Rinse the thermometer in cold water, dry it,
and stand it in antiseptic.

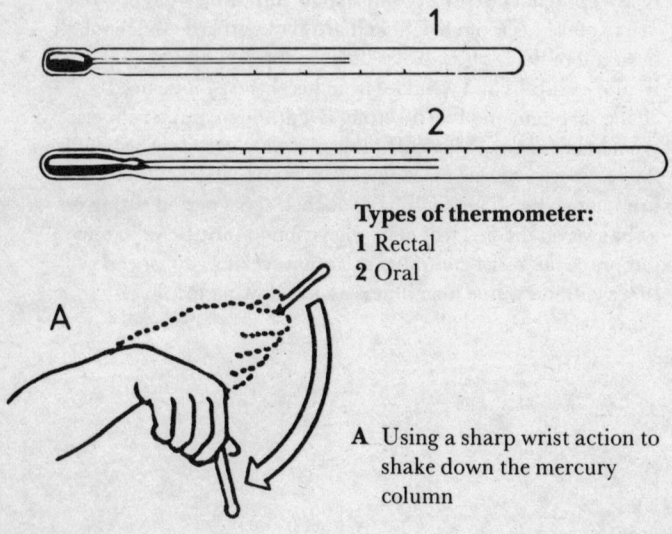

Types of thermometer:
1 Rectal
2 Oral

A Using a sharp wrist action to
shake down the mercury
column

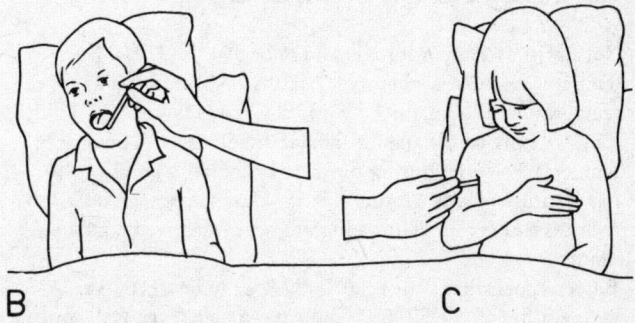

B Taking the temperature with
an oral thermometer in the mouth
C Taking the temperature with
a thermometer in the armpit

D Taking the temperature with
a rectal thermometer

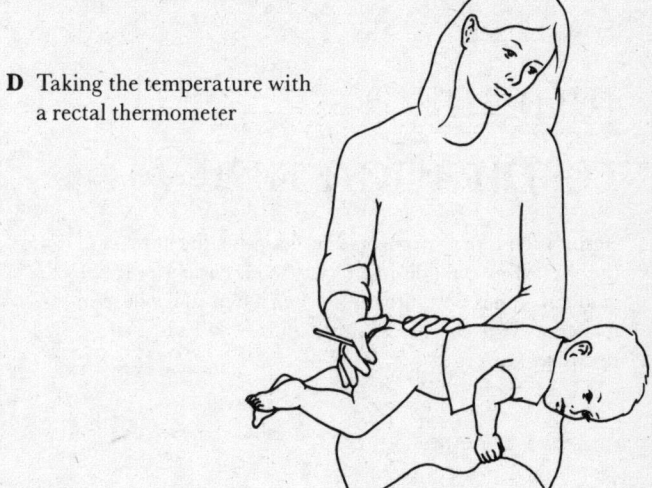

how to lower a temperature

Normal body temperature is said to be 98.6°F (37°C). But temperature fluctuates even in healthy bodies. In fact a temperature as high as 99.5°F (37.5°C) or as low as 97.7°F (36.5°C) may be normal for some individuals. Also body temperature varies during the day. Then, too, a child's temperature may be readily raised by excitement, an infant's by incessant crying. Thus a high temperature need not mean illness.

But a temperature above 100°F (37.8°C) indicates a fever. A temperature of 104°F (40°C) indicates a high fever. Call your doctor if the cause of a fever is not immediately obvious and manageable, and always in the case of a high fever.

To lower a child's temperature, give paediatric paracetamol, or, if prescribed by a doctor, aspirin. Also give plenty of water or fruit juice to drink. For high fever, the face and body may be sponged with tepid water to reduce the temperature.

judging a respiration rate

Respiration rate is discovered by counting the number of times the chest rises and falls in a minute. It is easily changed by emotion, and is best measured when a person is asleep or unaware of the check. Respiration rate, like pulse rate, decreases with age.

how to cope with vomiting

Vomiting can be due to motion sickness, obstruction of the digestive tract, food poisoning, indigestion, worry, tonsillitis, or infections, including scarlet fever. Attacks occur most often in early infancy. A vomiting attack is unpleasant to watch and can be frightening for the child. Deal with it calmly. Hold a bowl for the child and support him while the attack lasts. Then let him rinse his mouth with water. Wash his lips and face with a cloth. Change his bedclothes if they were soiled by the attack. Stay with him for a while in case he vomits again. Don't give him anything to drink for at least a couple of hours. Inform the doctor at once if the child is in pain.

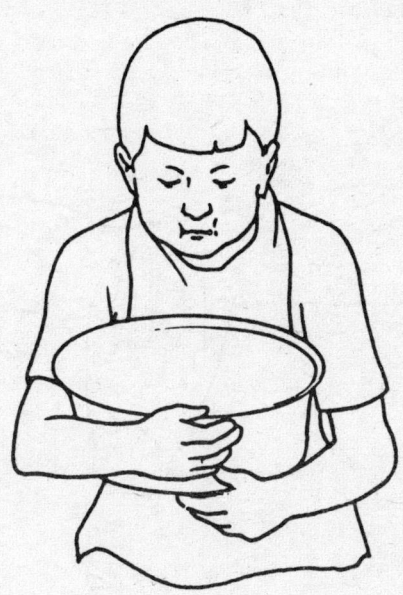

how to test the pulse rate

The heart's pumping action makes arteries expand and contract as blood pulses through them. Heart rate can be easily judged by finding the pulse rate of the artery in the wrist just below the thumb. To feel a patient's pulse, press your finger tips lightly but firmly on the wrist and move them gently until you feel the artery beating. Because the ball of the thumb has a pulse avoid using your thumb. The average pulse rate for an adult is 65–80 beats a minute. This increases with exertion, during infection, or under emotional stress. Children always have a high pulse rate. A baby's may be 120–140 per minute. A six-year-old child's may be 90. Pulse rhythm may vary as the child breathes in and out.

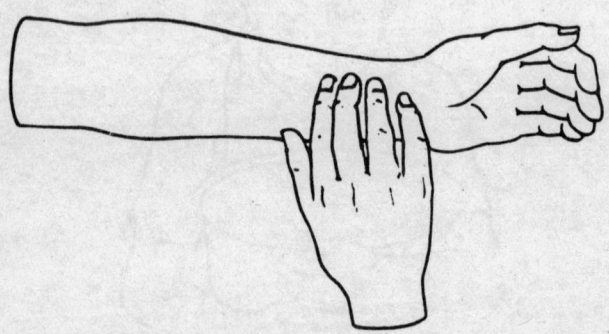

how to give medicine

Medicines can be dangerous if they are misused, and it is vital always to use them with care. Never give a medicine to anyone for whom it was not prescribed.

Points to remember
1 Adopt a matter of fact manner.
2 Check that it is the correct medicine – always preserve labels.
3 Check correct times of dosage.
4 Measure dose correctly.
5 Non-dissolving pills can be crushed and added to jam or honey.
6 Make a checklist of doses given.
7 Make sure bottle tops are always replaced securely.
8 Finish course if told to do so.

diet in illness

In many illnesses appetite drops off and some foods are not readily digested. Ask your doctor's advice on feeding if possible. The following hints are only general guides and some illnesses need special diets.

At the start of a high fever frequently offer water, soft drinks, and (if wanted) skimmed milk. In a day or two, if he is hungry, even a feverish child may cope with cereal, toast, soft-boiled egg, custard, ice cream, or plain biscuits. Children convalescing after a fever can usually tackle meat, fish, and vegetables.

After vomiting, wait two hours before allowing a sip of water. Later give half a glass, and, after several hours, a biscuit or a little cereal and some skimmed milk.

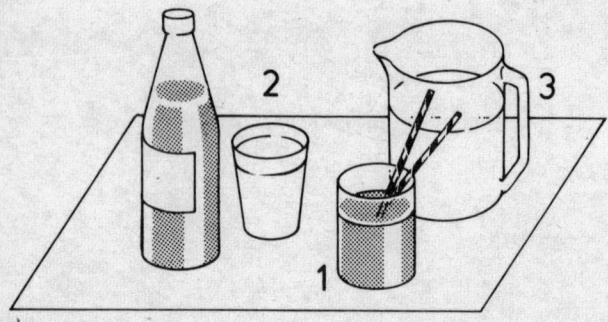

In simple colds, extra fluid may be helpful to children with diminished appetites.

In convalescence the child's appetite returns as he recovers. Meanwhile, forcing him to eat everyday foods before his digestive system is disease-free may cause revulsion and can even trigger long-term food fads.

Strict dietary rules apply to some medical conditions. Children with coeliac disease, for example, cannot absorb gluten and should not eat bread, cake, sausages, ice cream, or other foods that contain gluten.

Patients convalescing after a liver or kidney disease may need a high-protein diet. Adolescents need extra calcium for building bones.

Foods suitable for inclusion in the diet after one or two days of fever

1 Soft drink
2 Water
3 Skimmed milk
4 Cereal

5 Biscuits
6 Soft-boiled egg
7 Toast
8 Soup

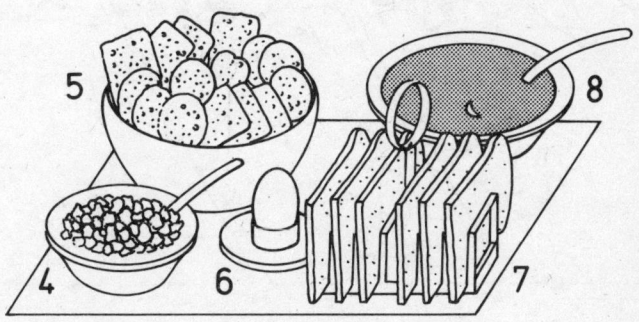

the sick child's progress

The progress of a child's sickness and recovery obviously varies with the type and degree of the illness. In general, however, a parent can expect the following.

1 Rest and sleep are among the most effective medicines for the really sick body. At this stage a child wants little more than a comfortable bed, a noise-free bedroom, and understanding.

2 When the child is well enough to sit up and eat meals, provide them on a tray, one course at a time, the food pre-cut if necessary. Make sure the food is tasty and attractive.

3 Early in his recovery a child prefers physically undemanding amusements: soft toys to hug; books or comics to glance at; a radio to listen to. His attention span may be brief.

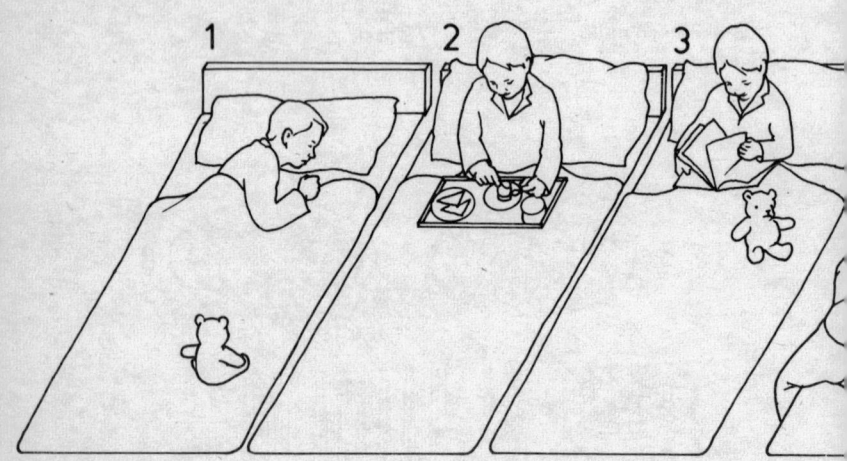

4 Convalescence can be boring for a child and visits cheer him up. But they should not be too long and the visitors should not be exposed to infection. If in doubt about the risk, ask a doctor.
5 A child on the way to recovery enjoys constructive, imaginative play: model making, sewing, making scrapbooks. It is more fun if you can help. Some schoolwork can be done in bed too.
6 When the child can get up for a time, he enjoys leaving his bedroom to watch television or sit with other family members. Make sure he is not in a draught. Use a blanket for warmth.

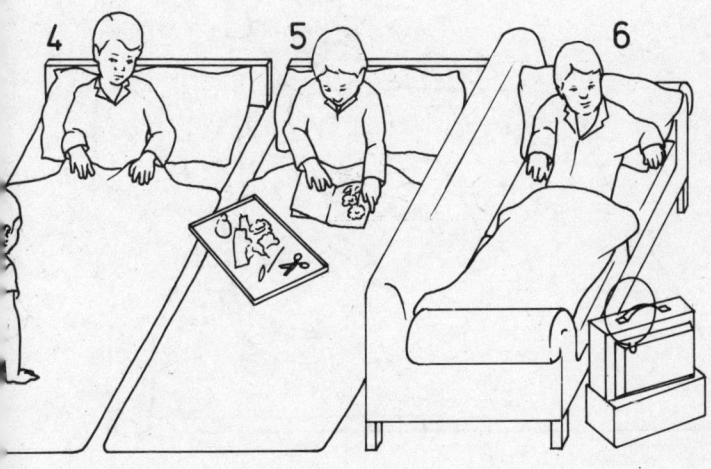

how to give a bed bath

The patient should be undressed and covered with a blanket. First wash face and neck, then arms and armpits. Roll the blanket to the waist and wash chest and belly. Cover the washed parts after drying thoroughly. Uncover one leg at a time and wash from feet to groin. Turn the patient on his side to wash his back. Let the patient wash whichever parts he is able to.

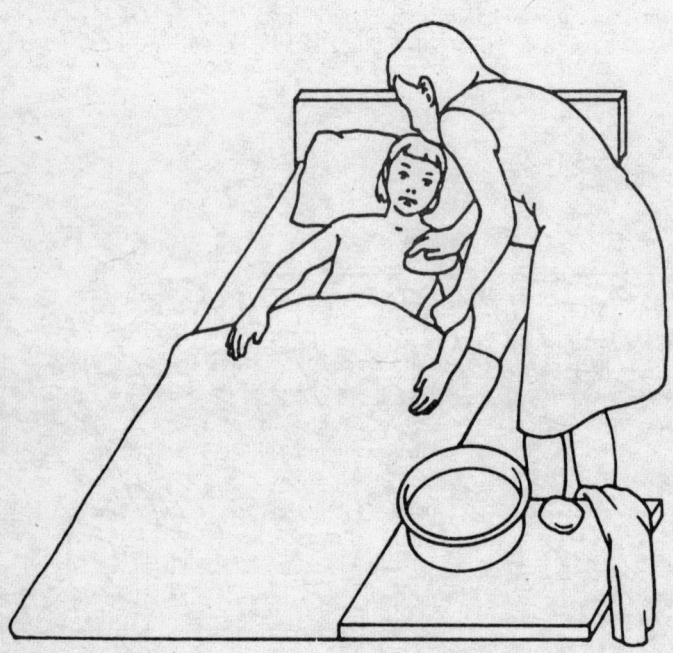

going to the hospital

Almost every child has to visit the hospital at some time, either as an outpatient, or for a longer stay for medical treatment or an operation. The unfamiliarity of the hospital and its staff, and the separation from his family, can make even the shortest visit a frightening experience for a child. Parents should therefore use every opportunity to familiarize the child with the idea of the hospital in advance by taking him there to visit a friend or relative. A simple explanation of the equipment that may be used and the treatment that he is likely to receive can be helpful, and a young child can be encouraged to 'act out' some aspects of the treatment on his toys.

outpatient visits

A short visit to a clinic or the hospital may be necessary for a variety of reasons.
Before admission to the hospital for surgical or medical treatment a visit to a specialist as an outpatient is usual.
Also, many routine tests or examinations and some minor surgical procedures are frequently performed in the outpatients' department.
The child should be warned in advance of his visit to the hospital, and, as in the case of an admission, he should be given some idea of what to expect.
A favourite book, toy, or game should be taken as delays between appointments are sometimes unavoidable even in the best-run department.

hospital admission

Admissions to the hospital fall into two broad categories –
routine and emergency.

Routine admissions

In the case of routine admissions the hospital admission is
arranged some time in advance – which has the incidental
advantage of giving the parents sufficient time and opportunity
to prepare the child.

Among children, the commonest reason for routine admission
to the hospital is for the correction of a congenital malformation
such as cleft palate or a faulty heart valve. Where possible,
doctors try to avoid admitting very young children to hospital,
but in some cases surgery has the best chance of success if it is
carried out at a particular stage of the child's development.

Emergency admissions

An emergency admission to the hospital is potentially more
disturbing for a child because of the lack of preparation time.
Perhaps the most useful thing that a parent can do to help in
these circumstances is to try to appear as calm as possible.
Reasons for emergency admission include the diagnosis of an
illness such as appendicitis that requires urgent treatment, or a
particular development in a disease that requires the child to
be kept under constant supervision.

An alarming number of emergency admissions among
children, however, are the result of accidents – many of which
could be avoided with better safety precautions at home and
outdoors.

hospital admission procedures

A thorough examination is customary when a child is admitted to the hospital. The child's weight, height, temperature, pulse, and blood pressure are normally recorded, and a urine test, blood test, and X-ray may be performed.

The parents will be asked routine questions about the child's earlier illnesses and previous visits to the hospital. This helps the doctor build up a general picture of the child's medical history.

If the child is to be admitted, he should be allowed to take with him a few favourite toys, and, if he has one, his security blanket. When the child undresses, it may be less alarming for him if his clothes are left nearby even if he cannot wear them.

hospital personnel

The children's department of a hospital is staffed with
personnel specially trained in child care.

The treatment of a child in the hospital is supervised either by
a paediatrician specializing in childhood disorders of every
kind, or by a specialist in a particular type of disorder.

Routine aspects of medical care and general welfare in a
paediatric department are the responsibility of the nursing
staff.

Where X-rays are needed, they will be studied by a radiologist.
Physiotherapists and occupational therapists may be involved
in the child's recuperation programme.

A dietitian, a play supervisor, and a teacher are now employed
in most paediatric departments, and a medical social worker is
usually available to discuss problems with both the child and
his family.

visiting your child

A hospital's visiting hours depend on its organization and staff arrangements.

In some hospitals visiting is normally allowed only at special times arranged to fit in with the daily routine of each department of the hospital. These restricted hours may make visiting difficult for some parents because of their hours of work or commitments at home, so many hospitals are now introducing unrestricted visiting in children's wards. This enables parents to visit at times that suit their particular circumstances.

A small child left alone in the hospital may feel frightened, overwhelmed, and even abandoned, and his loneliness and confusion may be reflected in a rather indifferent or sulky reaction to his parents' first visit. In general, visits should ideally be kept short and frequent, and parents should if possible use the time to play with their child.

A visit from brothers and sisters (if children are allowed as hospital visitors) will reassure a sick child and may also help the other children to become familiar with the hospital atmosphere.

Recognizing the severe emotional stress that a stay in the hospital can impose on a child, some hospitals now provide facilities for parents to remain with their child throughout his stay. If this is the case, a parent can help the child not just by playing with him and reading to him, but also by assisting in aspects of his day-to-day care such as bathing, changing clothes, and administering medicine.

Section 2:
ACCIDENTS

Introduction

Accidents are the most common cause of death among children. Every year all too many children are admitted to hospital, suffer serious disabilities, or die as a result of injuries caused by such accidents as falls, poisoning, or burns. Strange as it may seem, the majority of accidents happen in the home rather than outside. Pre-school children are particularly at risk from accidents in the home. A young baby may choke on food or a small object; an exploring toddler may fall down stairs, pull a scalding pan from the stove, swallow a household poison such as bleach, or even suffocate in a plastic bag. As a child grows older the type of risk changes: schoolchildren perhaps are more prone to accidents outside the home such as falls, swimming accidents and, of course, traffic accidents. Obviously not all childhood accidents are as serious as those already described. Minor cuts, bruises, and abrasions are part of the normal process of growing up and no amount of protection can ever prevent them. But even simple injuries can become emergencies and must be dealt with speedily and without panic. Every parent, apart from trying to risk-proof the home, must know how to deal with emergencies as they arise, be they a black eye or an electric shock.

The following pages provide a guide to some of the more common emergencies that can occur during childhood. They include minor injuries such as cuts, bruises, and abrasions as well as more serious injuries such as fractures, drowning, or burns. Also included is advice on when to call the doctor, ideas on the sort of first aid kit that every home should contain, and a guide to the most important first aid techniques such as bandaging, treatment of shock, and artificial respiration. Given a thorough training in these skills, any parent should be able to cope calmly and efficiently with any emergencies that happen to occur.

a basic first aid kit

Every home should have this home medical kit close at hand, in a box or metal container, and unlocked – but out of reach of children. It should be complete in itself – not dependent on kitchen scissors, for example. Its medicines and lotions should be clearly labelled, its dressings kept well wrapped. A basic first aid pamphlet (or copy of this book) and a notepad and pencil should be kept inside, and emergency phone numbers pasted to the lid. It should be sealed with adhesive tape, to keep it clean and dry and help keep out children. Similar kits should be kept in cars, boats, and caravans.

1 Adhesive tape
2 2½in bandage
3 1in bandage
4 An analgesic, eg paracetamol and paediatric paracetamol, or similar
5 Aspirin (for adults only unless prescribed by a doctor for a child)
6 Standard dressings
7 Scissors
8 Tweezers
9 Safety pins
10 Eyebath
11 Antihistamine cream
12 Antiseptic cream
13 Adhesive dressings
14 Petroleum jelly
15 Rubbing alcohol
16 Cotton wool

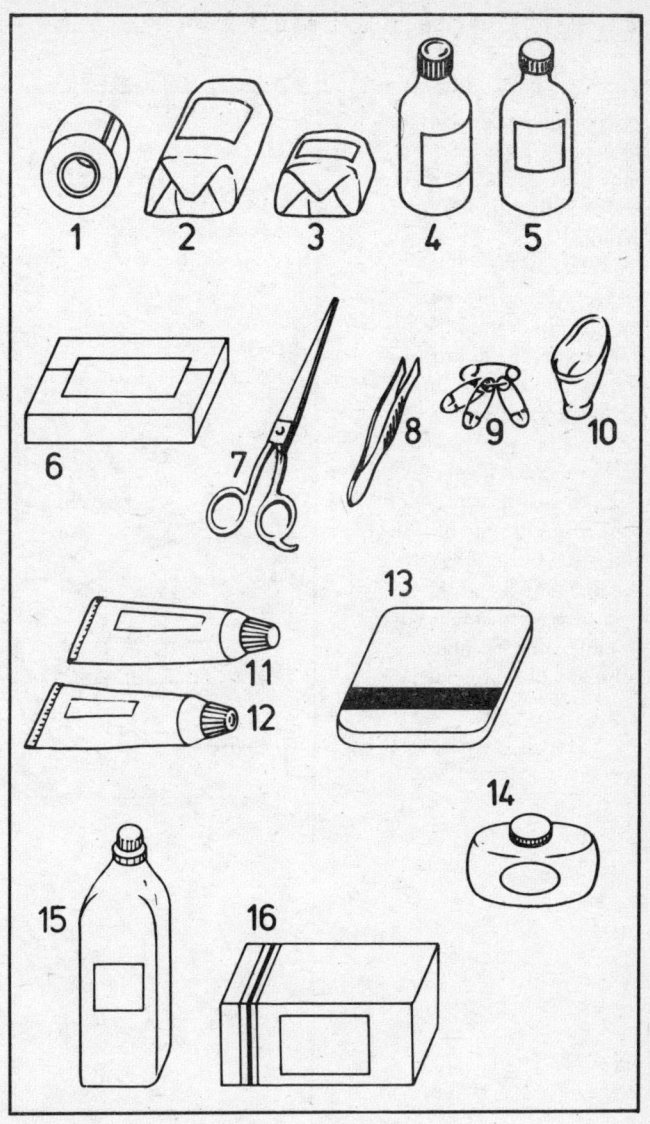

emergency items

Here are shown some common home articles that may be useful in an emergency. It is a good idea to have all of them near at hand.

Towels, handkerchiefs, and tissues are useful for cleaning or covering wounds. Vinegar may be applied to wasp stings, and bicarbonate of soda to other stings. Salt dissolved in water is a useful antiseptic. Salad oil may be used to float insects out of ears. A needle can be quickly sterilized by holding over a lighted match and then cooled before being used to remove splinters and superficially embedded stones.

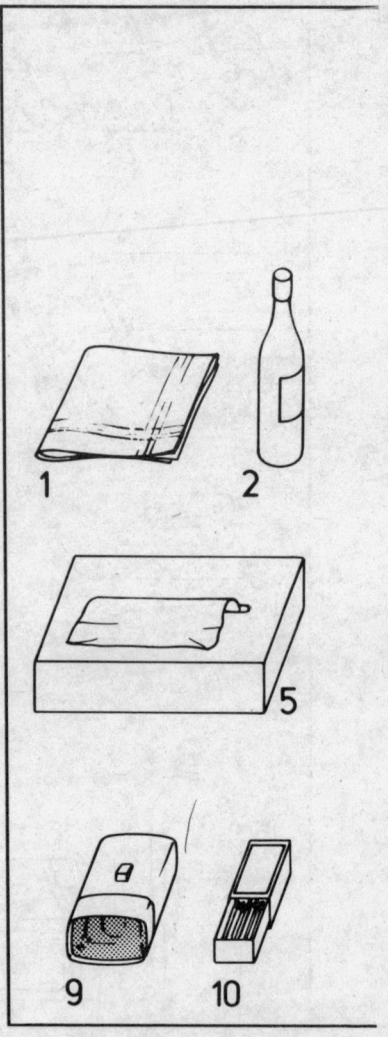

1 2

5

9 10

1 Handkerchief
2 Salad oil
3 Towel
4 Vinegar
5 Tissues
6 Salt

7 Packet of needles
8 Soap
9 Torch
10 Box of matches
11 Bowl of water
12 Bicarbonate of soda

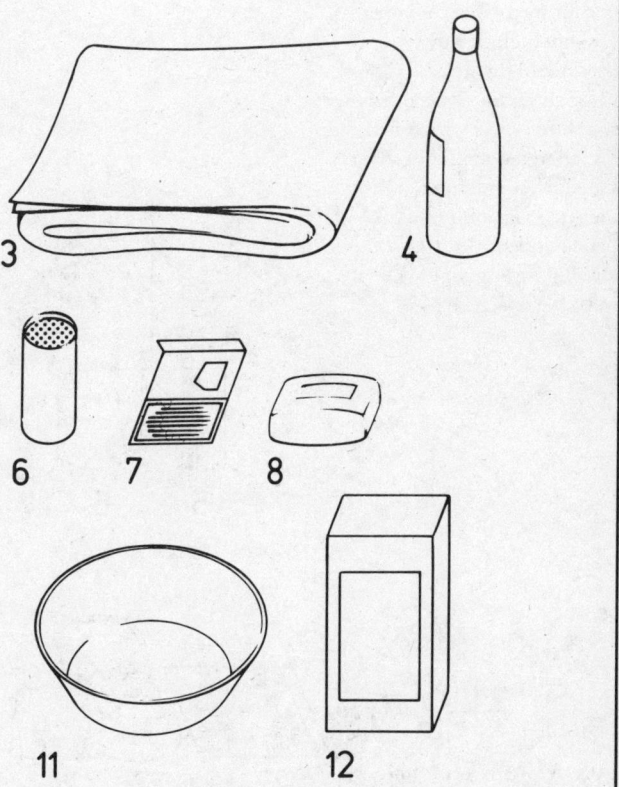

home treatment kit

This should have the contents of the first aid kit, plus additional items (mainly medicines and lotions). It can be divided into compartments: one for wound cleaning and dressing, one for bandages and instruments, one for medicines and creams. (Do not include any prescribed medicines, though: these should be locked away separately.) As with a first aid kit, all items should be clearly labelled and first aid instructions and notepad and pencil added. But you should still have a separate – more portable – kit, see p. 78.

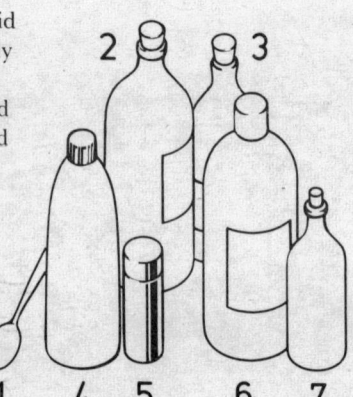

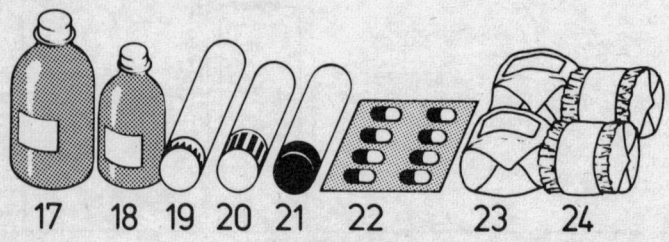

1 Dosage spoon
2 Cough medicine
3 Indigestion medicine
4 Diarrhoea remedy
5 Laxative
6 Calamine lotion
7 Toothache remedy
8 Scissors
9 Safety pins
10 Tweezers
11 Thermometers (oral and rectal)
12 Eyebath
13 Antiseptic cream
14 Antihistamine cream
15 Eye ointment
16 Eye drops
17 An analgesic, eg paracetamol and paediatric paracetamol
18 Aspirin (for adults only unless prescribed by a doctor for a child)
19 Throat tablets
20 Indigestion tablets
21 Motion sickness pills
22 Cold remedy
23 Bandages
24 Stretchable bandages
25 Triangular bandages
26 Gauze dressing
27 Cotton wool
28 Adhesive dressings
29 Adhesive tape

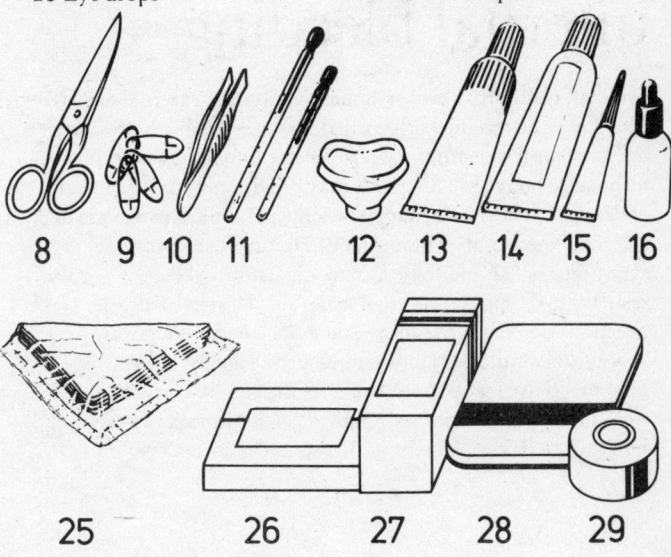

advice on wounds

In the case of wounds, get urgent medical help for:
a) any internal bleeding;
b) any external bleeding that will not stop;
c) a bleeding nose or ear after a blow on the head.
Keep the patient still, quiet, and lying down, and reassure him until help comes. Get medical aid without undue delay for:
a) any wound that has something embedded in it;
b) any puncture wound – one that is deeper than it is long (eg one made by a nail or knife point);
c) any wound from an animal bite;
d) any other wound that you think may be a tetanus risk (one that is deep and/or dirty).

internal bleeding

This can result from broken bones or ruptured internal organs. Blood may be coughed or vomited up, or be visible in the urine or faeces, or trickle from the nose or ear. Often, however, it is trapped in body tissues (which may swell) or in cavities like the abdomen of chest (which may become painful). In any case of internal bleeding the victim shows rapidly developing symptoms of 'shock' (pale face, cold, clammy skin, restlessness, rapid pulse, etc – see p. 93). Urgent medical attention is needed. Meantime take the measures against shock, and at intervals make notes for the doctor of the patient's pulse (see p. 64). Also note the colour of any blood from the mouth (bright red, frothy blood is probably from the lungs, dark red or black from the stomach, nose, or ear).

bruises and black eyes

A cold wet cloth on the damaged area will usually reduce pain and control swelling. This can be held in place if required with a bandage. Black eyes should be treated with care; if in doubt see a doctor – there may be eye damage or a concealed fracture.

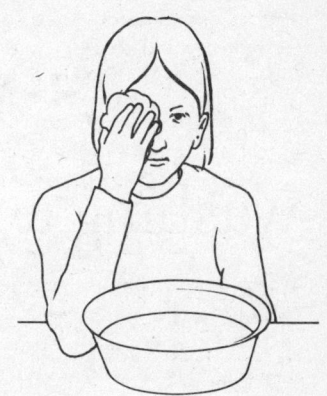

bleeding nose

Make the child sit quietly as shown, nostrils held pinched together. Tell him to breathe through the mouth, to let any saliva or blood dribble out into the bowl, and to avoid swallowing as this disturbs any blood clots that are forming. If after 10 minutes it is still bleeding, see a doctor. Slight nosebleeds are common in childhood, but see a doctor if they recur frequently.

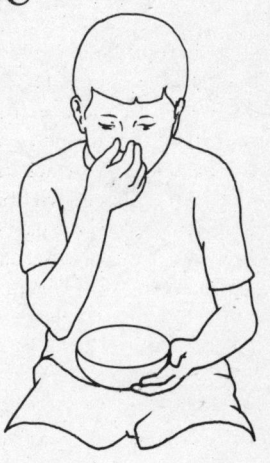

stopping bleeding

Press a pad of clean cloth against the wound (**1**). If bleeding
persists, add thicker cloths on top, and use more pressure.
Keep the injured area still, and calm the child. If a limb is
badly cut (but not broken), it helps to raise it above the level of
the rest of the body.

washing a wound

Wash your own hands first. Clean the skin around the wound
(wiping away from the wound), then the wound itself (**2**). Use
soap, running water, antiseptic (diluted according to the
instructions) and several fresh swabs of sterile gauze. Remove
all loose dirt, but leave any embedded matter for expert
attention.

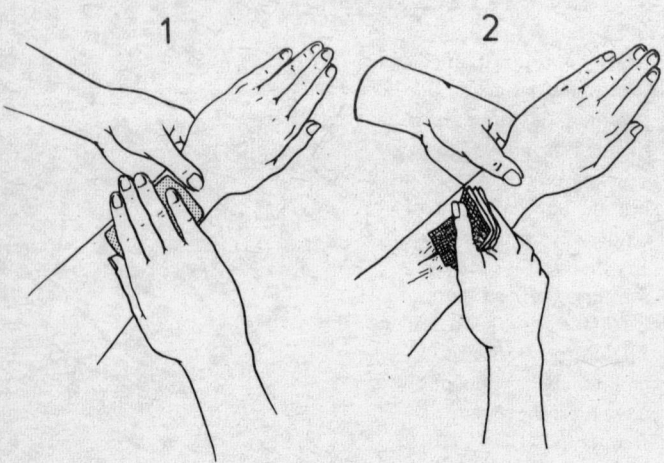

dressing a wound

Apply mild antiseptic, using sterile gauze. When dry, cover wound and surrounding skin with a piece of sterile gauze, handling it only by the corners. Put cotton wool on top, and keep this dressing in place with bandage or adhesive tape. Alternatively, use a prepacked sterile dressing and bandage. When bandaging, start at the narrowest point (**1**). Overlap the first few turns, then work up. Bandage firmly but not too tightly. Finish with a safety pin (**2**) or adhesive tape, or split and knot the bandage end. In an emergency, a clean handkerchief or other cloth can be used.

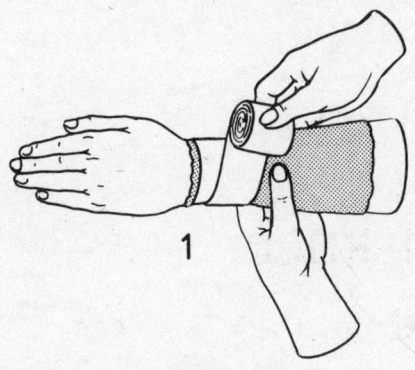

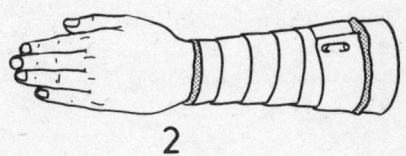

bandaging a finger

Use a sterile gauze as dressing, then cover with a long roll of narrow bandage. Run the bandage from base to tip of the finger, and back down the other side (**1**). Then wrap it around the finger (**2**), split the end (**3**), and tie (**4**). A finger stocking (**5**) helps keep the bandage clean and secure.

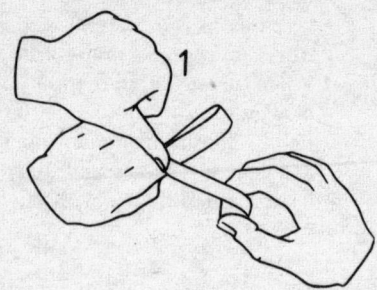

elbow or knee bandage

Place the bandage against the elbow (or knee), point upwards (**1**). Then wrap one of the bottom ends around the joint (**2**), and repeat with the other bottom end (**3**). Tie these two ends together, not too tightly (**4**), and finish by tucking the bandage point down over the knot (**5**).

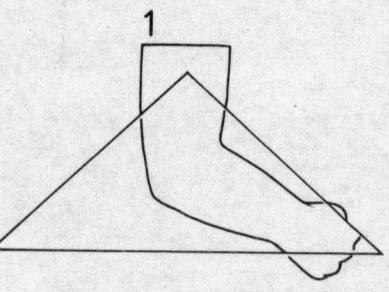

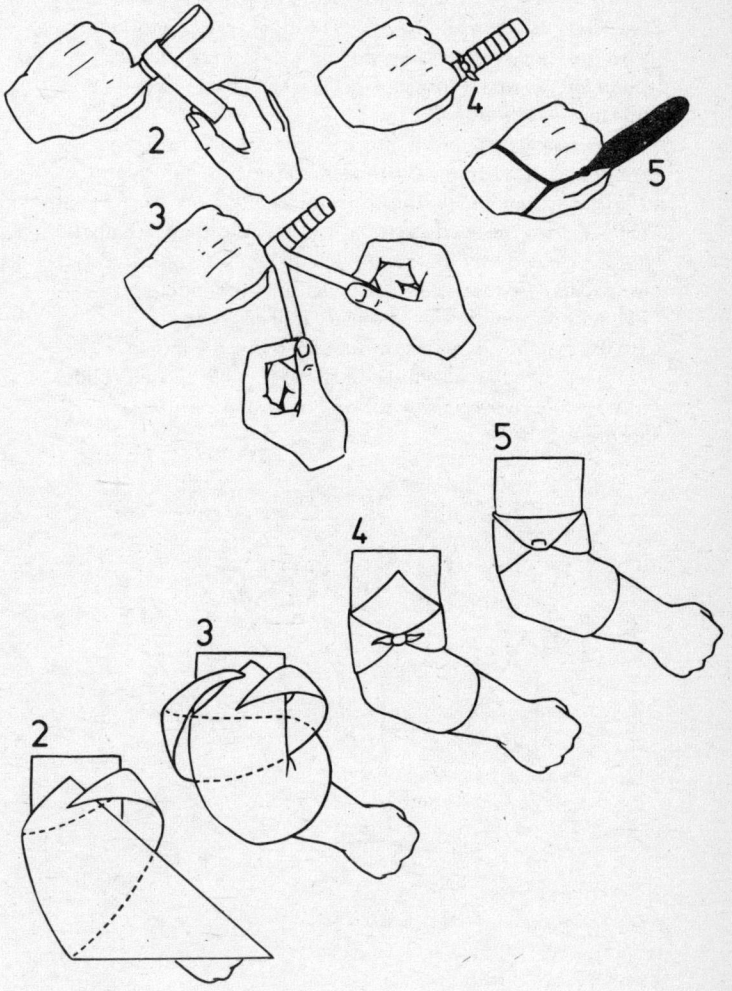

artificial respiration

Mouth-to-mouth respiration is the most commonly used form
of resuscitation and can be used in almost any case where
breathing has stopped. This may occur because of smothering,
drowning, electric shock, or inhaling gas. If there are any
bystanders, send one for help, and start artificial respiration
immediately as follows.

a) If necessary turn the victim on to his back and turn the head
to one side, clearing any debris from the mouth (**1**).

b) With one hand under the neck and the other on the crown of
the head, turn the head as far back as possible, then pull up the
chin to the head until it is fully tilted up (**2**). This position
ensures that the tongue does not obstruct the windpipe.

c) Open your mouth wide and place it firmly over the
casualty's mouth, pinch his nostrils, and breathe into his
mouth, enough to make his chest rise (**3**). (With a small child,
put your mouth over his mouth and nose, and use quicker,
shorter breaths.)

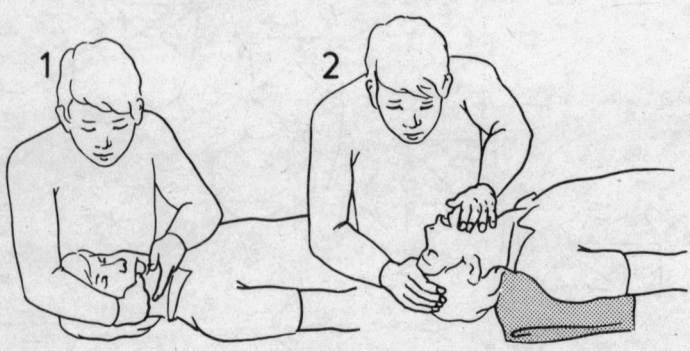

d) Remove your mouth and watch the chest fall (**4**), then repeat once every 3 seconds for children (once every 5–6 seconds for adults).

e) If the chest does not rise, check the victim's head and chin position, and that his tongue is not blocking the back of his throat.

f) If still unsuccessful, put the casualty's head down for a moment over your lap, and slap him sharply between the shoulder blades to dislodge any blockage. Wipe the mouth clear.

g) Don't give up till the victim starts to breathe. Many have revived after hours of artificial respiration.

h) When he is breathing strongly, keep him warm and get help. Don't let him get up. Put him in the recovery position (see p. 92) if you think he may vomit.

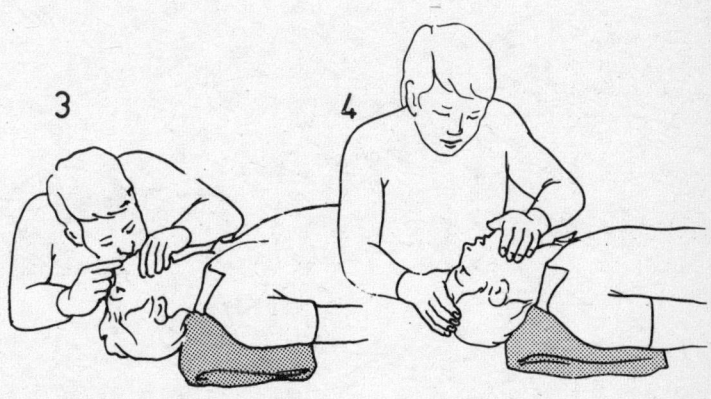

recovery position

Death following unconsciousness is often the result of the tongue blocking the airway or the casualty inhaling his own saliva or vomit. Provided that there is no possibility of neck or spinal injury, persons who are unconscious but breathing should be placed in the recovery position shown: with stomach down; head turned to one side; and arm and leg on that side pulled up till the thigh is at right angles to the body, and the hand level with the jaw. Pull the chin forward and up, so that the tongue cannot block the throat. Loosen clothing around the neck, and see that the mouth is clear of debris, blood, or mucus. Do not put a pillow under the head. In fact, if possible, raise the legs and body slightly above head level, so fluids drain away from the lungs. Look for hidden bleeding beneath clothes or body; deal with any external wounds. Then cover with one blanket and watch closely till help comes. Give nothing to drink even if consciousness returns.

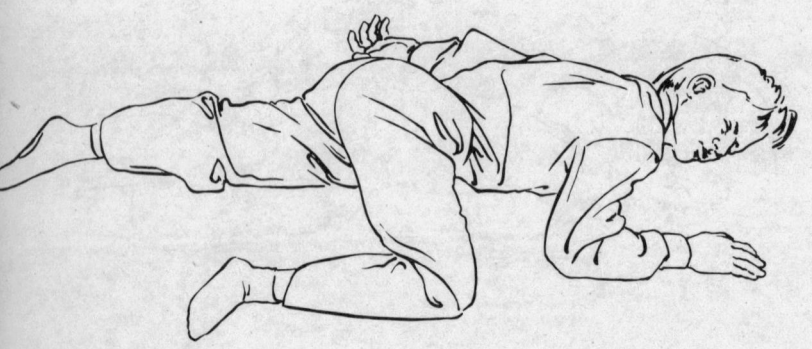

treating shock

Shock is of two kinds:
a) nervous shock, due to emotional trauma or severe pain; and
b) surgical shock, due to loss of body fluid (eg from bleeding, burns, or repeated vomiting or diarrhoea).
The second is much more dangerous. The victim is pale, with a cold or clammy skin, or rapid pulse, and rapid, shallow breathing. He is often restless or apprehensive, with nausea and thirst. He may faint. You should act quickly.
1) Lay the casualty down. Use the recovery position if vomiting seems likely. Otherwise lay him on his back with his head low and his legs raised if possible.
2) Deal with the physical cause of shock (eg try to stop any bleeding).
3) Get medical help.
You can also loosen the patient's clothing at neck, chest, and waist, and cover him with a sheet or thin blanket. Moisten his lips if he is thirsty, and if possible note his pulse and breathing rates. Do not:
a) warm the patient (but do retain body heat, eg with a blanket)
b) move him unless forced to;
c) give him anything to drink until he has been seen by a doctor.

treating an electric shock

Act fast – every second counts.

1) Break the victim's contact with the current in the quickest SAFE way (see below).

2) Check his breathing, and use artificial respiration if necessary (continue for hours if need be: recovery is still possible).

3) If breathing but unconscious, put in recovery position (see p. 92).

4) Give first aid to any burns.

5) Get help urgently.

Breaking electric contact

a) Pull out plug, turn off current at fuse box, or pull away appliance by cord; or

b) pull at a DRY, LOOSE part of the victim's clothing; or

c) push or pull at the body with any dry non-metallic object.

But DO NOT touch the victim's body; and be sure you are standing on a dry surface and touching only dry materials.

coping with an epileptic fit

In a fit the victim seems jerked by uncontrollable spasms. His head may be thrown back, his lips turn blue, his eyes roll up, his mouth froths. Do not try to restrain him, or throw cold water over him, or pick him up to rush for help. But do guide his movements, remove furniture, and lay him on the ground so that he cannot hurt himself. If the casualty's temperature is raised (check for facial flushing) loosen his clothing to reduce it. Also keep his airway clear by loosening clothing at the neck and turning his head to one side so saliva drains out. If you can, guide him into the recovery position (see p. 92). A fit usually lasts only a few minutes. Afterwards, put him to bed and get medical advice. Give no food or drink.

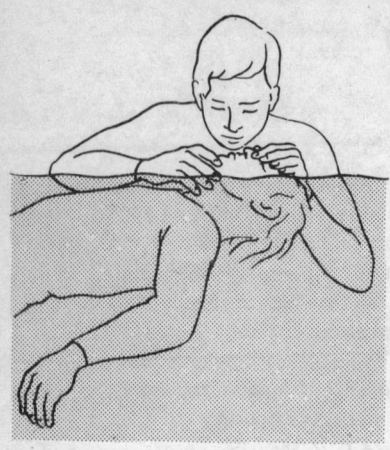

drowning

Start artificial respiration (pp. 90–91) at the earliest safe moment (eg in shallow water, in a boat, or at the water's edge). Do not try to drain water from the lungs; any that comes up will probably be from the stomach. Just clear the mouth of water, seaweed, etc, and give artificial respiration till breathing starts.

fainting

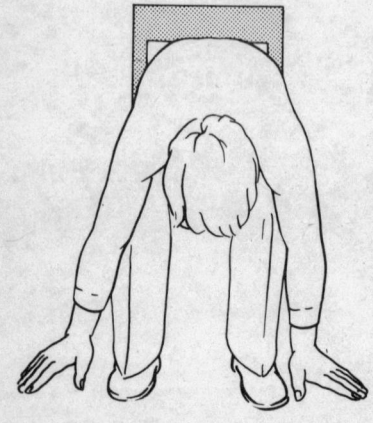

If someone feels faint, make him lie down or sit as shown, and breathe deeply till he feels better. If he faints, lay him down on his back, head low, legs raised. Loosen tight clothing (especially at the neck), and let him come round in his own time. If the fainting lasts more than a minute or two, keep him warm and get medical attention.

choking

Choking is always a potential emergency. If it occurs, put the child over your knee or over a chair back; or, if he is small enough, pick him up bodily. Then give three or four firm slaps between the shoulder blades. If this does not work, get medical help at once, and give artificial respiration (pp. 90–91) if necessary. Two other possible courses of action may cause serious injury and should be tried only as last resorts – reaching into the throat and trying to extract the object, and the so-called Heimlich technique. For the latter, for older children only, stand behind the child with your fists clasped above his abdomen, then push them up hard towards you.

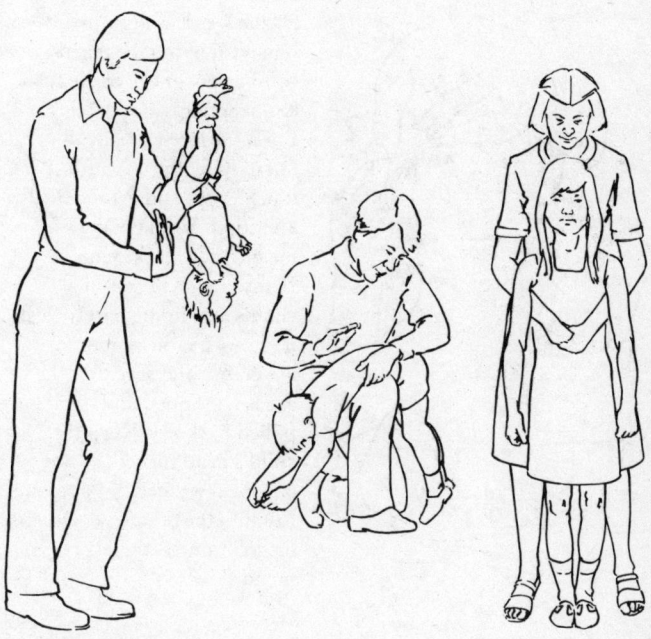

foreign body in the eye

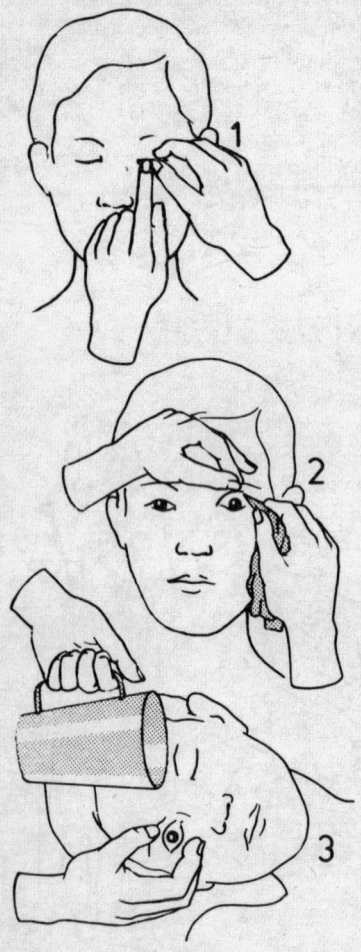

Stop the child from rubbing the eye. If the object is sharp or hot, or if the eye is bleeding, do nothing, but get medical attention at once. But if it is probably just a speck of dust, bring the upper eyelid down over the lower, as shown (**1**) while the child turns his eye upward, or wash the eye, using an eyebath or eyedropper. If these fail, look for the speck, and try to remove it with moistened cotton wool or the corner of a handkerchief (**2**).

But if the foreign body does not move with the gentlest touch, stop, and get medical attention. Bandage the eye meanwhile to ease pain.

If any chemical gets in a child's eye, immediately flush it out with large amounts of water, making sure that the eye is wide open and the lids pulled back (**3**). Keep the child's head turned, so any chemical washed out does not run into the other eye. Do this for 15 minutes, then get medical help.

foreign body swallowed

If the object is smooth, small, and rounded, it should cause no trouble. Just give normal diet, and examine the child's bowel movements for a few days, to make sure that the object has passed through. See a doctor, though, if the child is under two, or if he seems to become unwell. But if the object is sharp or pointed; or if there is any chance that it might have been inhaled into the lungs, not swallowed; then give nothing to eat or drink, and get medical help.

removing splinters

If the splinter protrudes, wash your hands, wash the area well, and pluck out the splinter with sterilized tweezers or needle point. Press the skin so that a spot of blood comes from the wound, then wash well or apply a mild antiseptic. Cover with sterile dressing if necessary. Deeply embedded splinters or inflamed wounds need medical attention.

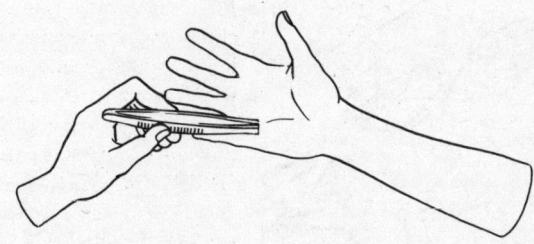

removing rings

Rings can get stuck because they are too small, or because the finger has swollen due to injury or infection. Smearing the finger liberally with soap (**1**) may allow the ring to be pulled off. If not, try binding thread tightly around the finger (**2**) for a short distance above the ring. Pull the ring up onto the bound part, unwind the thread behind it, and bind again above where the ring now is. Continue until you have worked the ring off the finger. But do not leave the binding on for any length of time, or else the blood supply to the finger will be affected.

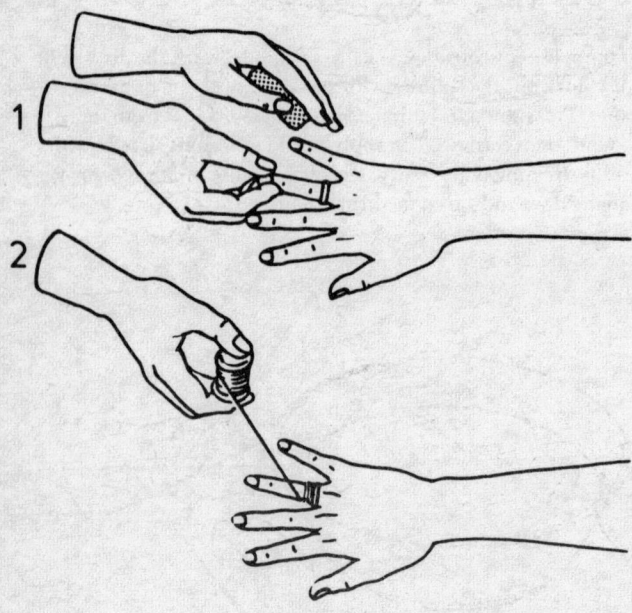

looking after grazes

Remove any loose dirt, etc, with moist sterile swabs, or with tweezers sterilized in boiling water for five minutes. Then treat as a wound (p. 87). But do not try to get out anything that is stuck or embedded; just wash the surrounding area, dry, put on a sterile dressing, and get medical attention.

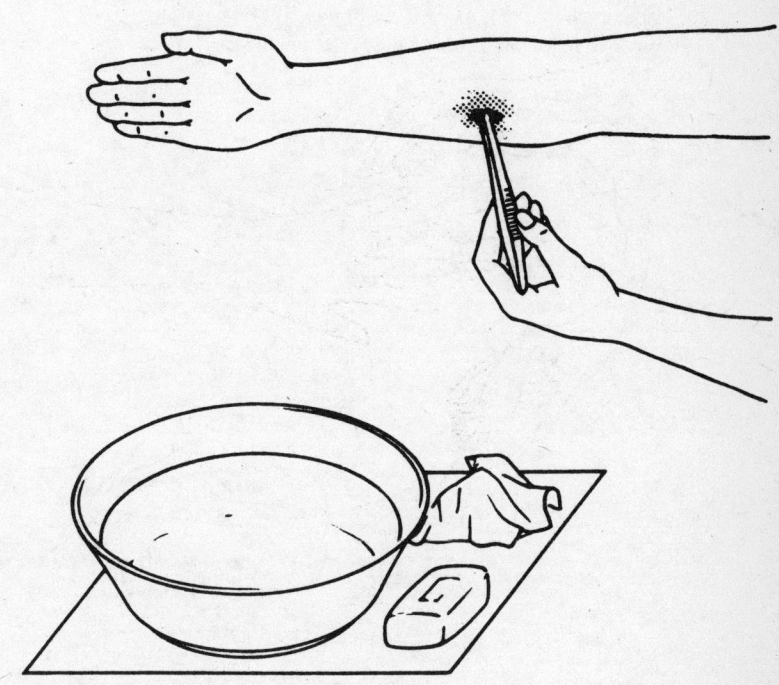

foreign body in the nose or ear

Foreign body in the nose
If the object is small and smooth, a sneeze will usually dislodge it: use pepper to set off sneezing (**1**). If this does not work, get medical advice. Do not try violent nose-blowing, or probe into the nostril, or squirt any water or oil into the nose.

Foreign body in the ear
If the child has an insect in his ear, put in a few drops of lukewarm olive or mineral oil. This will stop the frightening buzzing, and may even wash the insect out. However, with any other object in the ear, do nothing, except to tilt the head to one side, as shown (**2**), to see if the object falls out. If not, get medical help; any probing may damage the ear.

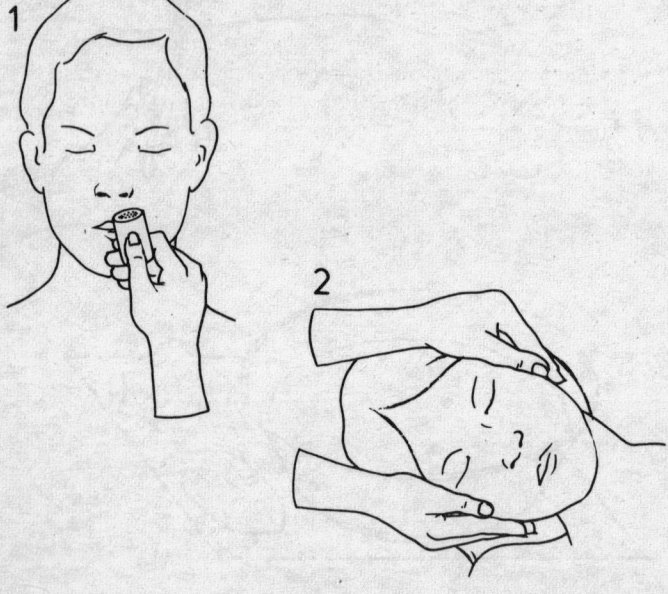

items that can contain poisons

Most homes are full of poisonous items that can only too easily be eaten or drunk by a child. Some of the most common items are listed here.

1) Some household chemicals, eg insecticide, rat poison, and weedkiller; paraffin, petrol, turpentine, and any cleaning fluid; liquid furniture and car polish; and alkalis used for cleaning drains, bowls, etc; oil of wintergreen, ammonia, bleach, sodium carbonate, and detergents; mothballs, and lead-based paint (which should never be used on indoor surfaces).

2) Some toiletry articles, eg perfume, cosmetics, hair tonics, nail polish and remover.

3) Many prescription and some non-prescription drugs.

4) Alcohol.

5) Food containing bacteria; and misused food (eg salt given to a baby in mistake for sugar).

6) Some common house plants (and water they stand in), eg oleander, dieffenbachia, poinsettia, and garden plants, eg ivy (the berries), laburnum (the seed pods), deadly nightshade and the foxglove.

helping a
poisoned child

Some common signs of poisoning are shown on the illustration below. If you suspect your child has swallowed poison you must act quickly.

Possible signs
1 Unconsciousness
Unusual sleepiness
2 Very red face
3 Mouth burns
Vomiting
4 Convulsions
Rapid, deep breathing
5 Stomach pains
Diarrhoea

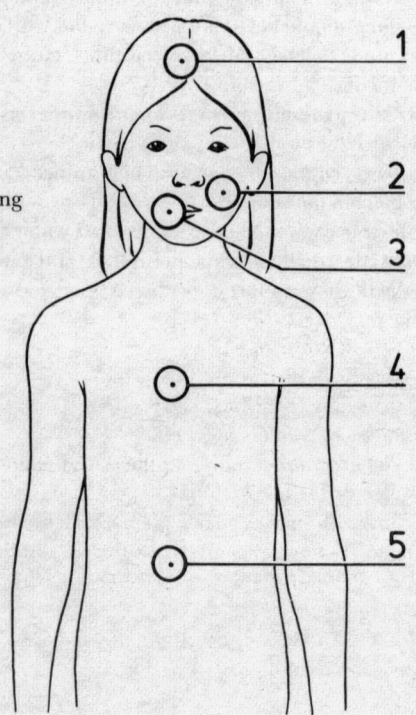

1) If breathing is failing, give artificial respiration (see pp. 90–91).
(NB: use mouth-to-nose respiration if there is any chance of poison still in the mouth.)
2) If breathing but unconscious, put in recovery position (see p. 92).
3) If conscious but likely to vomit, put in recovery position (see p. 92).
4) Question the victim, if possible, and look for evidence of the poison (empty bottles, scattered pills, an odour, pills in mouth).
5) Call emergency help.
6) Decide whether to make the patient vomit: see below.
7) Keep the patient warm till help comes. Do not leave.
8) Keep a sample of the poison and any vomit.
Still get attention even if: the patient vomits, and then seems all right; the poison seems to have had no effect; you are not sure if any poison was taken.

Induced vomiting
Make the patient vomit ONLY if:
a) he is fully conscious; and
b) he is not convulsing; and
c) you know for certain that the poison is not an acid, alkali, or liquid petroleum product.
To induce vomiting, tickle the back of the throat with your fingers. Before he vomits make the patient lie on his front, with his head lower than his body and over a bowl. Induce repeated vomiting if possible.
If it is safe to induce vomiting, it is also safe to give bland fluid (eg water or milk) afterwards to dilute any remaining poison.

bites and stings

Animal bites

Animals and plants can also be a source of hazard for children. In the case of animal bites, calm the victim. Use running water on the wound to flush out saliva. Then wash wound well for five minutes with sterile swabs, using soap and water (not strong antiseptics such as iodine). Rinse, dry, and dress the wound. Animal bites are seldom serious, but always seek medical advice. Anti-tetanus injections may be needed and the doctor may also recommend injections against rabies.

Snake bites

The most important first aid is to reassure the casualty and keep him calm and very still, preferably lying down. Flush the wound with soapy water and wash away any venom that remains around the bite or oozes from it. Support and immobilize the affected limb, for instance by splinting it, and obtain medical help as soon as possible. If the casualty's breathing begins to fail, start artificial respiration.

Fleas, lice, ticks

Isolated lice and ticks can be loosened by covering them with oil, grease, turpentine, or nail polish. They can then be removed with tweezers (with ticks make sure that you remove the head as well as the body). Crush the creature, and flush away or burn. Clean flea, louse, or tick wounds with soap and water or a mild antiseptic, and apply calamine lotion or antihistamine cream. (For treatment of infestations of fleas and lice, see p. 48.)

Bees, wasps, hornets

If the sting is still in the skin, scrape it out with a sterilized needle. (Do not pull it out with tweezers or fingernails: you may squeeze more poison into the wound.) If the sting has just occurred, apply antihistamine cream. If not, run cold water over the area, dry the skin gently, and then apply a solution of bicarbonate of soda. For a sting in the mouth, give a mouthwash of bicarbonate of soda solution, and give ice to suck. Get medical help if:

a) the victim shows signs of general distress, eg skin rash, pallor, weakness, nausea, or tightness in chest, nose, or throat;
b) there is a dangerous swelling (eg from a sting in the mouth);
c) the victim has been stung many times; or
d) there is a history of allergy to stings.

Mosquitoes, gnats, ants

Wash with soap and water. Apply calamine lotion, antihistamine cream, or a paste of bicarbonate of soda and water. Cover any swelling with a cold wet cloth. Do not let the child scratch the bite – this can damage the skin and increases the risk of infection.

Mosquitoes and gnats can carry disease so if any complications develop within a few days get medical advice, especially if in a tropical or subtropical country.

Jellyfish stings

Treat with calamine lotion or antihistamine cream. But if the victim gets short of breath, or faints, get emergency medical attention.

types of burn

There are three main types:
1) dry burns, caused by fire, over-hot material (eg metal or rubber), electricity, or friction;
2) scalds, caused by over-hot liquid including oil or steam; and
3) chemical burns, caused by acids, alkalis, and some other chemicals.

1 Dry burn
2 Scald
3 Chemical burn

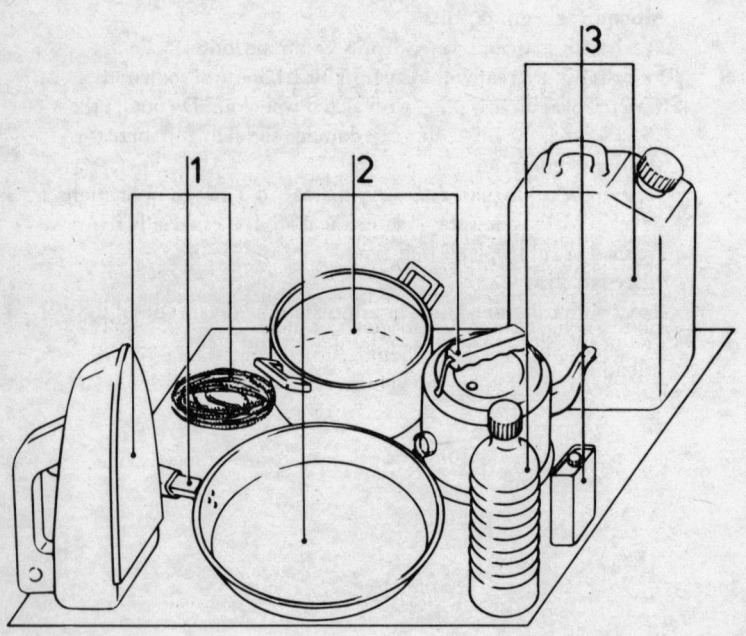

the seriousness
of a burn

This depends on its area and depth. The area will be obvious.
Degrees of depth include:
a) skin reddened, but not blistered;
b) skin blistered;
c) layers of skin destroyed.
The first two are 'superficial', the last 'deep'.
Any deep burn, however small, needs medical attention. But a
large superficial burn can be more dangerous, for shock due to
loss of body fluid (see p. 93) depends on the area of a burn, not
its depth. Pain is no guide to a burn's seriousness: a deep burn
can destroy nerve ends, so no pain is felt.

chemical burns

Chemical burns are caused by acids (eg hydrochloric acid),
alkalis (eg caustic soda), and some other chemicals. With
chemical burns, always wash the burn with large amounts of
water for up to 10 minutes. If the injury is slight, remove any
affected clothing, using gloves if necessary. If the injury is
severe, this is even more important as clothing will be soaked
with the chemical; remove clothing as quickly as possible, but
very carefully so that the flesh underneath is not damaged.
Then treat as for non-chemical burns (see pp. 110–111).

treatment of burns

Treatment of superficial burns

Small superficial burns (ie smaller than the size of the victim's palm) should be treated in the following way. Run cold water over the burn for a few minutes (**1**). Wash own hands well; also wash the burn gently if dirty. Dry the burn. If there is no blistering of the skin, a mild, soothing ointment may be applied. If there is blistering, apply nothing, and do not pierce the blisters, simply cover the burn with a sterile non-fluffy dressing and bandage (**2**).

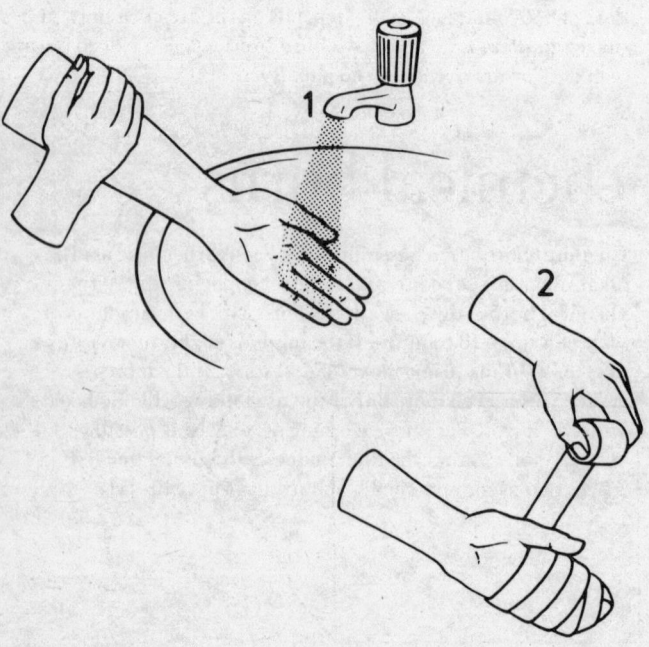

Treatment of other burns

Run cold water over the burn for at least 10 minutes. Apply nothing except a dressing, give liquid if the child is conscious, and then send immediately for medical attention. Do not breathe on the burn or touch it, and do not pull away clothing stuck to it. If large areas are involved, also give treatment for shock (p. 93), and get help urgently. With very large burns, immerse till help arrives (**3**).

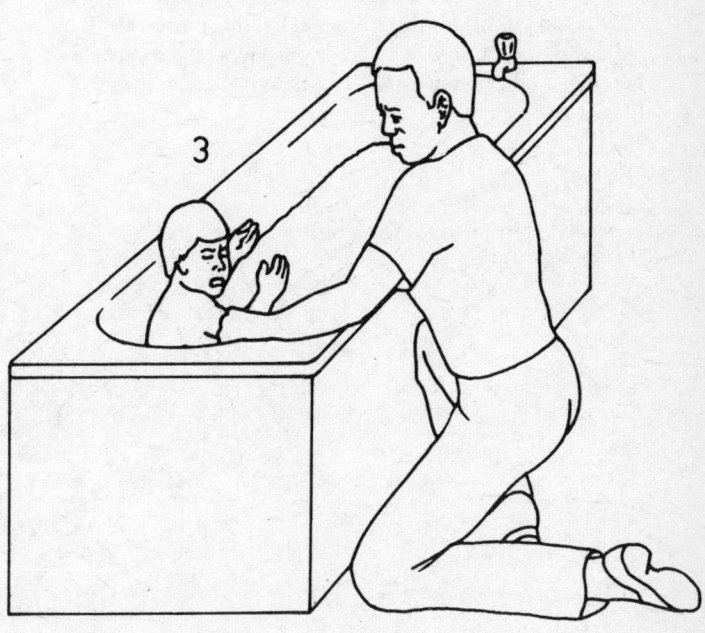

treating heat and sun effects

Heat exhaustion

This develops gradually in very hot and humid conditions, when the body sweats profusely. Loss of body fluid and salt produces shock. Symptoms include muscle cramps, exhaustion, restlessness, a pale face, and cold, clammy skin. Often there is dizziness, headache, nausea, loss of appetite, rapid breathing, and a rapid pulse. Make the victim lie down in a cool, darkened area, fan air over him, and apply wet cloths to the head and body. Get him to drink a glass of water containing ½ teaspoon of salt, and repeat this three times at half-hour intervals. If the child is young, or does not recover quickly, get medical help. If fainting or unconsciousness occur, treat immediately as heatstroke.

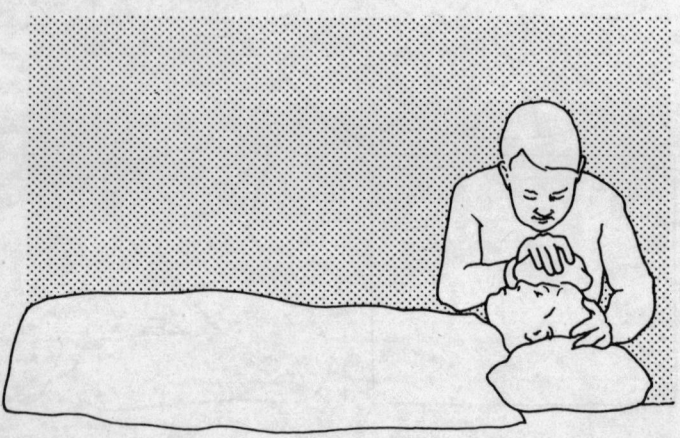

Heatstroke

This is similar to heat exhaustion but more sudden and severe. The victim is red-faced, with hot, dry skin and a high temperature (eg 104°F:40°C). Breathing is noisy, the pulse strong but fast. Stupor or unconsciousness is common. The urgent need is to get the body temperature down. Strip the victim, and immerse in cold water – or keep pouring cold water over him. Once his temperature is below 102°F (38.8°C), wrap the child in cold, wet sheets in the recovery position (p. 92). Fan air over him. Get medical help.

Sunburn

Treat as a burn. If there is no blistering and the burned area is small, apply ointment or lotion. If more severe, apply only a sterile dressing, and get medical advice.

treating effects
of extreme cold

Frostbite

Warm the victim gradually at room temperature, and give
warm food and drink (not alcohol). Thaw out the frostbitten
parts slowly: eg cover frostbitten ears or nose with a gloved
hand, place frostbitten fingers in the armpits under the
clothing. Do not apply heat directly to the frostbitten part, or
rub it, or immerse it in hot water, or apply snow. Finally, begin
to move the frostbitten part very gently. Get medical attention.

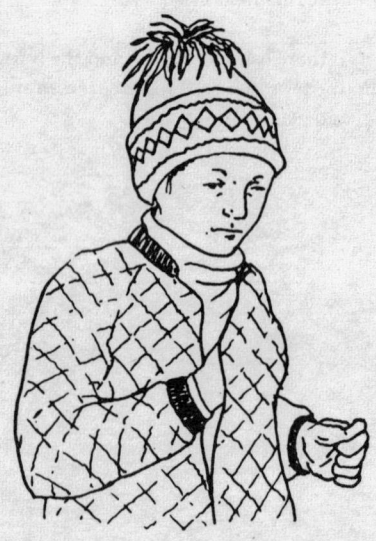

Frostbite: warming frostbitten fingers in armpit.

Exposure

Remove wet clothing, wrap the victim in dry blankets, and get him to warm conditions. If possible, place him in a bath of warm water (not too hot). Dry, place in a warm bed, give warm drinks, and get medical help.

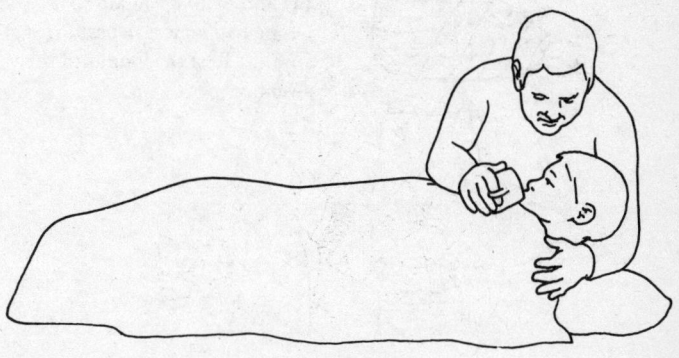

Exposure: giving warm drinks.

sprains

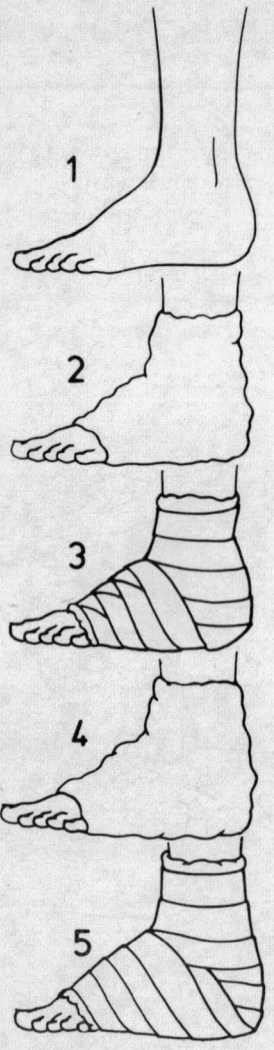

An active child may suffer a number of joint or muscle problems. Sprained ankles are common. The ligaments of the joint are stretched or torn, causing swelling and pain, which increase if the foot is used. A cold compress may reduce the swelling, and firm bandaging may relieve pain, but it is best to get medical attention as well in case of fracture. To bandage, surround the joint (**1**) with a thick layer of cotton wool (**2**) and then bandage firmly as shown (**3**). On top, apply a second layer of cotton wool (**4**) and bandage again (**5**). Crepe bandages are best for sprains. Rest the foot until the swelling goes down.

pulled muscles

This is overstretching or tearing of muscle fibre, due to a sudden movement or to handling heavy weights. There is a sudden sharp pain, then pain whenever the damaged part is moved. Make the victim comfortable, with the injured part supported, and get medical attention.

cramp

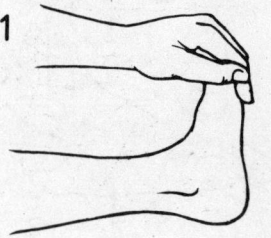

This is sudden painful contraction of a muscle, brought on by chilling (as in swimming), or badly coordinated movement, constriction, or loss of salt and body fluid (eg through sweating). If it occurs, treatment involves forcibly contracting the opposite set of muscles, so that those causing trouble relax by reflex. The drawings show correct procedures for cramp in the foot or calf (**1**) and hand (**2**).

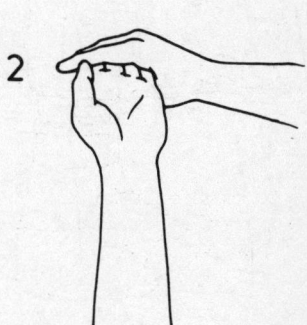

dislocation

The joint is immovable and very painful, and looks deformed.
Do not use force, or try to put the bone back in place. Support
the limb in a comfortable position (a dislocated leg can be
bound to the good leg, in a lying position). Get medical
attention. Watch the limb for impaired circulation.

1 Normal joint
2 Dislocated joint
3 Sign of dislocation

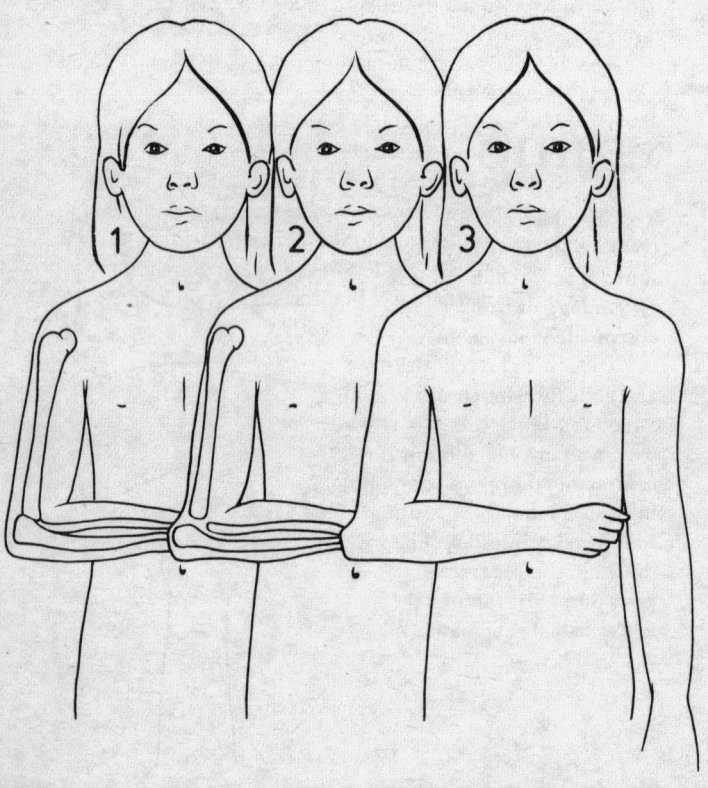

fractures

Childhood fractures sometimes go unnoticed and untreated.
This can be because a child's nervous system may not register
the pain very acutely. Also children's fractures are often
'greenstick' ones, with no complete break in the bone. So watch
the child for other signs of a fracture: tenderness, swelling,
and bruising. A broken limb is also often misshapen and
uncontrollable. If you do suspect a fracture:
(a) do not let the child use or move the affected part, and do not
move or straighten it yourself;
(b) stop any bleeding (see p. 86), and lightly cover any
protruding bone with sterile dressings;
(c) keep the child warm, and treat for shock if necessary; and
(d) get medical help.
Do not try to push a protruding bone back in, or clean its
wound. And do not move the child, except to avoid further
immediate danger – in which case use a stretcher. Moving
someone with a broken neck or back is especially dangerous.
The only exceptions to the rule about moving are for a broken
wrist, arm, or collarbone, when you can move the child to
transport or to a warm place. But first support the arm well
with a sling.

types of fracture

The main types are: (**1**) closed – the skin surface is not broken;
(**2**) open – the bone is exposed to the air (ie it protrudes, or
there is a deep wound over it);
(**3**) 'greenstick' – the bone is bent or not completely broken;
(**4**) splintered – part of the bone is shattered;
(**5**) complicated – some other part of the body (eg a blood
vessel, or a nerve) has also been damaged in the fracture.

1 Closed   **2** Open   **3** Greenstick

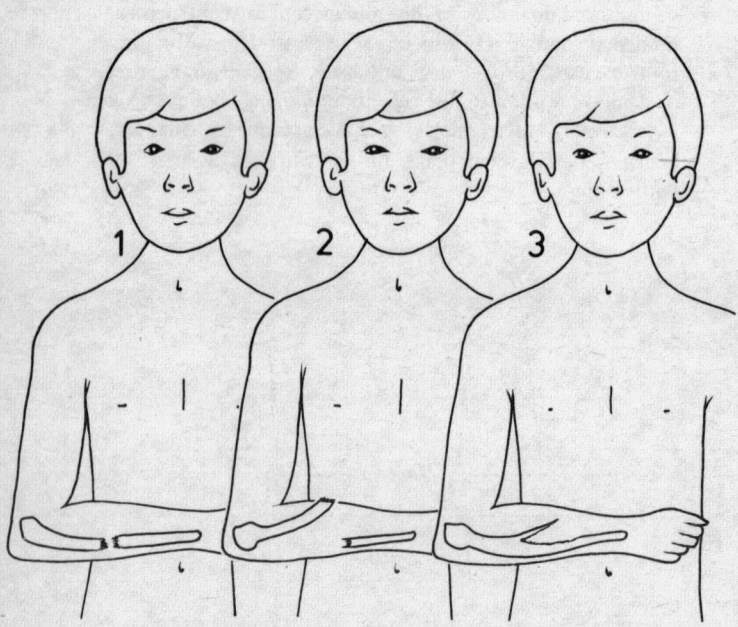

making a splint

A splint is used to immobilize a broken limb, if medical help is not quickly available. Wood, metal, or stiffly rolled newspaper can be used, and the splint is bound to the limb above and below the break with padding in between, firmly but not too tightly. Alternatively, a broken leg can be bound to the good leg to steady it, and a broken arm to the chest.

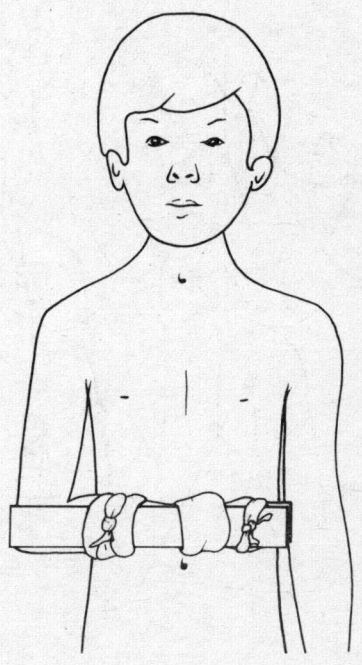

making an arm sling

Using a triangular bandage:
1 put the bandage between the chest and forearm, with the point out beyond the elbow and the top round behind the neck;
2 bring the bottom up in front, tie to the top, and fasten in the point.

Improvising a sling
Improvised slings can be made with belts, scarves, neckties, or pinned-up sleeves.

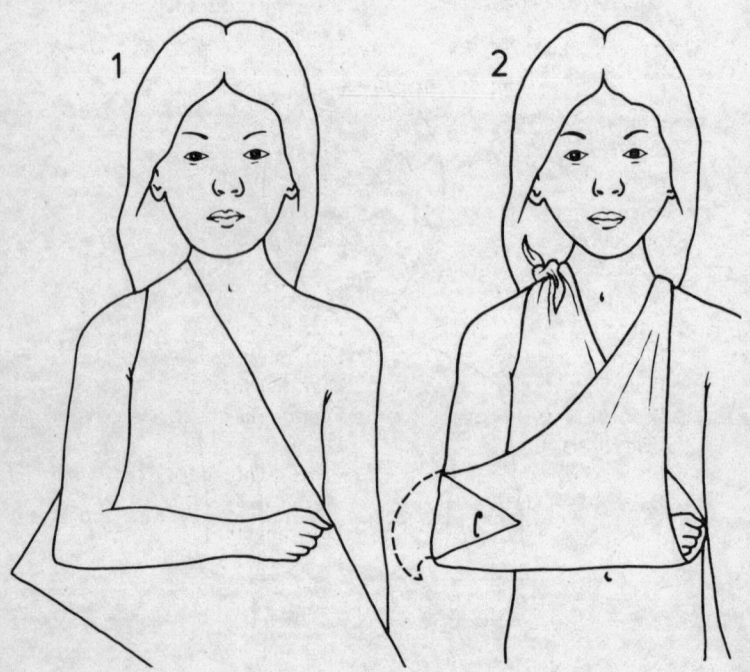

INDEX

EMERGENCY INDEX

A SELECTED LIST OF NON-FICTION TITLES AVAILABLE FROM CORGI BOOKS

THE PRICES SHOWN BELOW WERE CORRECT AT THE TIME OF GOING TO PRESS (MAY '86). HOWEVER TRANSWORLD PUBLISHERS RESERVE THE RIGHT TO SHOW NEW RETAIL PRICES ON COVERS WHICH MAY DIFFER FROM THOSE PREVIOUSLY ADVERTISED IN THE TEXT OR ELSEWHERE.

☐ 12697 7	**Beating Your Heart**		*Richard Adler*	£1.95
☐ 12257 2	**The New Book of First Names**		*Michele Brown*	£2.95
☐ 12706 X	**Good Children**		*Lynette Burrows*	£2.50
☐ 12820 1	**Drugwatch: Just Say No**	*Sarah Caplin & Shaun Woodward*		£1.95
☐ 10336 5	**The Magic of Honey**		*Barbara Cartland*	£1.50
☐ 12718 3	**Life Without Tranquillisers**		*Vernon Coleman*	£2.95
☐ 12742 6	**Dad's Baby**		*Diagram Visual Info. Ltd.*	£2.95
☐ 12741 8	**Child Development**		*Diagram Visual Info. Ltd.*	£2.95
☐ 12740 X	**The Parent's Emergency Guide**		*Diagram Visual Info. Ltd.*	£2.95
☐ 12735 3	**The Fix**		*Brian Freemantle*	£2.95
☐ 12379 X	**Judith Hann's Total Health Plan**		*Judith Hann*	£1.75
☐ 12480 X	**Hayfever: No Need to Suffer**			
		Colin Johnson & Dr. Arabella Melville		£2.50

All these books are available at your bookshop or newsagent, or can be ordered direct from the publisher. Just tick the titles you want and fill in the form below.

Transworld Publishers, Cash Sales Department, 61–63 Uxbridge Road, Ealing, London, W5 5SA

Please send a cheque or postal order, not cash. All cheques and postal orders must be in £ sterling and made payable to Transworld Publishers Ltd.
Please allow cost of book(s) plus the following for postage and packing:

U.K./Republic of Ireland Customers:
Orders in excess of £5; no charge
Orders under £5; add 50p

Overseas Customers:
All orders; add £1.50

NAME (Block Letters) ....

ADDRESS ....

....